THE
SOUTH CAROLINA
STATE
HOSPITAL

THE
SOUTH CAROLINA
STATE
HOSPITAL

Stories from Bull Street

WILLIAM BUCHHEIT

THE
History
PRESS

Published by The History Press
Charleston, SC
www.historypress.com

First published 2020

Manufactured in the United States

ISBN 9781467144728

Library of Congress Control Number: 2019951251

For my late cousin Heather, who spent so much of her life caring for others.

CONTENTS

ACKNOWLEDGEMENTS

First, I'd like to thank the twenty-four men and women whose stories are featured in this book. They spent hours answering my questions and telling me about their lives, and most of them were able to scrounge up old photos to personalize their stories.

I also owe a great amount of appreciation to those who provided information about the South Carolina State Hospital and put me in contact with people to interview: Jan Bob Barkow, Ginny Caldwell, Jonathan Cochran, John R. Edwards, Sarah Lewis, Lorry May, Kay McCrary, Jane Westbury and South Carolina's mental health commissioner, Gregory Pearce.

Obviously, this book would not have been possible without the help of the South Carolina Department of Mental Health (SCDMH), its employees and its archives. I'm particularly indebted to SCDMH's public information director, Tracy Lapointe, for her encouragement and for helping me gain clearance to photograph the campus in 2010 and 2011. I'd also like to thank the National Alliance on Mental Illness (NAMI), especially South Carolina's chapter, for awarding me Reporter of the Year in 2011. Without such advocacy groups, the mentally ill wouldn't have a voice at all. My gratitude also goes out to the *Aiken Standard* newspaper for its stellar coverage of the SCDMH and state hospital during the second half of the twentieth century.

My genuine thanks goes out to The History Press and its editor Chad Rhoad for agreeing to publish this book.

I, no doubt, owe a degree of debt to photographer Christopher Payne. It was, after all, his photobook *Asylum: Inside the Closed World of State Mental Hospitals* that sparked my interest in the decline of mental institutions and the displacement of their patients.

As family members go, I owe thanks to my brother Phil for giving me photography pointers in my early days of exploring and shooting the Bull Street campus.

I also owe credit to my sister Bonnie and mother, Mellnee, for their continued love and support during the long process of writing this book. I'm grateful as well to my aunt Brenda for giving me firsthand accounts of her visits to the hospital to see a patient in the late 1960s.

Lastly, I want to thank all the former South Carolina State Hospital patients who contacted me with their own stories of life on Bull Street. Your help was essential to my study of the iconic institution, and it helped me better understand all the institution's strengths and shortcomings.

INTRODUCTION

I n early 2010, I was ambling through a Barnes & Noble when a large photobook caught my eye. Under the cover's image of a dangling straitjacket screamed the title in red capital letters: *ASYLUM: INSIDE THE CLOSED WORLD OF STATE MENTAL HOSPITALS.*[1]

The second I opened the book, I was captivated. Its creator, New York photographer Christopher Payne, had visited dozens of abandoned state hospitals across America, shooting both the interiors and exteriors of the castle-like structures.

Perhaps the most illuminating facet of Payne's work is its assertion that these institutions did a lot more than treat and house the mentally ill. In essence, they functioned as self-sustaining communities with their own greenhouses, slaughterhouses, bowling alleys, dairies, stables, laundries, cemeteries and full-service medical facilities. However, the thing I found most interesting about *Asylum* was the way it provided a visual history of psychiatric treatment in our country. Most of the hospitals Payne photographed have been reasonably well preserved and remain intact; anyone who tours the hospitals is transported to a bygone era when the colossal structures pulsed and howled with the afflicted.

Asylum did more than spark my curiosity and imagination, it created a yearning in me to see and photograph one of these old mental hospitals firsthand. The asylum closest to my house in Upstate South Carolina is the South Carolina State Hospital in downtown Columbia. It was a sprawling

180-acre property that was tucked away from the general public for nearly two centuries. Known statewide as "Bull Street" because its entrance lies at the corner of Bull and Elmwood, the South Carolina State Hospital is the nation's second-oldest public mental facility, admitting its first patient in 1828.[2]

Even though I'd lived within a mile of the institution as a graduate student from 1998 to 2001, I'd never once been inside its gates. All that changed on Superbowl Sunday 2010, when I drove through the campus on my way back home from a bachelor party in Charleston. It was a cold, wet afternoon, and since I had no game plan at the time, I drove toward the single-level structures at the rear of the property. Eventually, I parked my car behind the Saunders Building, where it would be less visible, and grabbed my camera. A few minutes later, I was scouring the back porch of Saunders when I discovered a door that had been propped open. With my heart hammering against my sternum, I pushed the door forward and squeezed through the opening to get inside.

The Saints and Colts were just hours away from kicking off the Superbowl, but it's hard to imagine that any of the players were as excited and nervous as I was inside those unfamiliar surroundings. Perspiration stung my scalp as I inhaled the musty air and gazed at the thick strips of paint peeling off the walls. It was clear the building hadn't functioned as a hospital for at least a decade, because there was little in the way of artifacts to be found. Yet, the darkness, silence and decay trapped inside the building had an inescapable allure. I thought about the prospects of ghosts, security guards and homeless people finding me inside, but most of all, I wondered about what had taken place in the hospital when it flowed with life.

Over the next eighteen months, I returned nearly two dozen times to explore and photograph the decaying hospital's campus. Along the way, my interest in Bull Street went from abstract curiosity to undeniable obsession. As many hours as I spent creeping through the menacing darkness of the hospital, I spent just as many off campus researching the institution's history. I found it stunning how little had been written about the hospital and continued to think about all the lives that had been saved, changed and lost there.

During those years of research, I was still working full time for a chain of newspapers in Spartanburg, and I thought it might be interesting to write a series on Bull Street. Who better to tell the story of the hospital, I figured, than the men and women who'd worked there? So, I spoke with employees of the South Carolina Department of Mental Health

(SCDMH) and asked if they could point me toward any interesting interviewees. Most people gave me the same name: Woody Harris. Around Columbia, Harris had earned a reputation as the state hospital's unofficial historian. As you will read in the first chapter of this book, the interview did not disappoint. Over a couple hours at his house, Harris relayed stories about the good, bad and ugly things that he'd witnessed during his long career at Bull Street. "To me, it was the world's most interesting place," he explained.

Before I left that afternoon, I asked Harris to recommend other former employees to interview. He took a deep breath and said, "Elbert and Gertrude Metze." The Metzes are the only people in this book who worked at the state hospital during the first half of the twentieth century. Although they were in their late eighties when I met them in 2010, I found them remarkably lucid when it came to describing their respective careers at Bull Street. I interviewed two more subjects that year: former hospital director of budgeting Jack Balling and its former chief psychologist Dr. Jack Luadzers. Both revealed critical details about the deinstitutionalization movement that swept through the hospital in the 1980s and 1990s and ultimately led to its demise.

That four-part news series led me to a closer examination of the current state of mental healthcare in South Carolina, which I quickly learned was deplorable. After publishing several stories on the failures of the system the following year, I slowly gained the attention of advocacy groups around the state. In 2011, I was awarded the Reporter of the Year award by the South Carolina chapter of the National Alliance on Mental Illness (NAMI). I received the honor at a NAMI banquet at the Embassy Suites in Columbia, and to this day, it remains the most treasured award of my career.

Despite this positive recognition, as 2012 arrived, the Bull Street project went cold. The only story I would write that year would be that of Rachel Bricco, a retired nurse from Greenville who had worked in the state hospital's Byrnes building in the mid-1980s. The following year (2013), I again wrote one state hospital story, which was that of Tom Summers, who had served as the institution's chaplain for four decades. Apart from those articles, it appeared as if my sources from the hospital had dried up. No matter how many times I spoke to locals and SCDMH employees, I just could not find another former state hospital employee to interview. For more than a half decade, I ceased writing about and photographing the institution, and I felt content moving on to the next chapter of my life. But after a temporary move to Charleston for another job, I returned to Greenville and contemplated resuming the state hospital project. My recent business endeavor had taught me the power of social media advertising, and I promptly took out a Facebook advertisement to locate potential subjects. It read, "I am compiling a book of people's memories of the old Bull St. hospital in Columbia. If you ever worked or visited there, I'd love to talk to you." I also created a Facebook page named "SC State Hospital Book," where I posted some of the stories I'd written and photos I'd taken from 2010 to 2012.

To my delight, my advertisement garnered responses almost immediately. One of the first people to contact me was Linda McLamb, who worked at Bull Street during the summer of 1961 as a student nurse. Hers was a harrowing and horrifying tale about one of the more difficult periods in the hospital's history. McLamb spared few details as she recounted the overcrowding, understaffing, neglect and hopelessness she observed while working in the Saunders building. The retired nurse even gave a vivid account of seeing a patient days after she'd received a lobotomy, the much-demonized brain surgery that historians have claimed was never performed on the Bull Street campus. My story on McLamb, which ran on May 23, 2018, in the *Greer Citizen*, signified my full-fledged return to the project after five years.

It also rekindled my journalistic fire and restored my hope that I'd one day have enough stories for a book. When I posted the story on Facebook, it garnered a substantial response, especially from those in the Midlands. After that article was published on social media, my search for subjects became easier, and I was able to interview at least one former state hospital employee every week of the summer in 2018.

At first, it was mostly nurses who contacted me, and boy, did they have some stories to tell. In their stories, they described their experiences with suicides, patient attacks, electroshock therapy and virtually every conceivable mental disorder known to man. In addition, they told me how it was usually their job to administer medication, update records and share vital information with patients; after all, as any former Bull Street employee can attest, most of the psychiatrists who worked there in the second half of the twentieth century were immigrants who didn't speak English very well. Because of this, nurses were also usually the highest-ranking mental health workers with whom patients could talk.

Gradually, I did manage to achieve some diversity in my subjects— something I considered essential to any comprehensive study of the hospital.

Public safety officers Phil Parker and Sam Alexander worked to keep the peace when patients or staff members got out of hand. Volunteer Robin Stancik spent half a decade entertaining schizophrenic women whose families had dropped them off on Bull Street, never to return. Activity therapists Loretta Smith and Kim Grant, meanwhile, designed recreational projects and off-campus field trips so patients could actually have some fun. Social workers at the state hospital also played a critical role in patient treatment. John McMaster (the current governor's older brother) worked with patients who'd been ruled not guilty of crimes by reason of insanity. After he helped mold that unit into one of the best of its kind in any U.S. state hospital, McMaster spearheaded Bull Street's employee assistance program and became the primary counselor to hundreds of the hospital's employees. Melton Francis, meanwhile, began working in the admission wards of the hospital after he earned a master's degree in social work from the University of South Carolina in 1977. During his eighteen months at Bull Street, he witnessed the inherent problems of deinstitutionalization and watched a revolving door of patients go through the hospital.

Though this book primarily focuses on the stories of those who worked at the state hospital, there are a few exceptions. The first of these is the chapter on Carol Hall-Martin and her brother, Richard Hall. Those two fine people are the only living children of the iconic William S. Hall, who served as state hospital superintendent for two decades before becoming South Carolina's first mental health commissioner in the 1960s. During his career, which lasted for nearly five decades, Hall relentlessly campaigned for more state dollars to be allotted toward mental health, as his hospital was consistently one of the three most underfunded public psychiatric institutions in the nation. Hall's love for Bull Street, its patients and its staff is documented in this book through the vivid memories of his children. Then, I've included the story of one brave patient: Jan Wise. Though, over the years, I've spoken to more than a few people who were committed to the institution, most of them preferred to remain anonymous, and it isn't hard to see why. Even as the third decade of this new century dawns, mental illness continues to carry a heavy stigma in American culture. Yet, from the moment I first spoke with her, Jan Wise wanted to tell her story, without the protection of anonymity, in order help others like her, who are facing major psychiatric disorders. Wise was committed to Bull Street soon after her second suicide attempt in 1982, and she credits a doctor there with helping her get back on her feet. Not only did her stay at Bull Street return her to functionality, it allowed her to flourish, earn a degree in psychology and dedicate her life to helping children—first at the South Carolina Department of Juvenile Justice (DJJ) and then at the Boys and Girls Club of the Midlands.

IN TWENTIETH-CENTURY AMERICAN CULTURE, the state hospital became a symbol of captivity, horror and chaos. Indeed, the prospect of losing one's freedom is terrifying enough, but the thought of losing one's mind along with it is too grim for most souls to entertain. Hollywood's portrayal of the state hospital as some kind of hell on earth full of sadistic doctors, mean nurses, shackles, straightjackets and icepick lobotomies did not ease these fears. Such stories and films left a mark on our collective perceptions that is as glaring and irreversible as a surgical scar.

Human beings fear the unknown, and most Americans have never seen the inside of a state hospital. In writing this book and telling the stories of these special men and women, I hope to illustrate the iconic Bull Street institution as a place that not only did a lot of good but also served a critical purpose. Throughout the second half of the twentieth century, the South Carolina State Hospital housed, fed and treated thousands of patients who were incapable of surviving on their own. When it was first introduced, the community care model of psychiatric treatment that was designed to replace the state hospital model sounded good enough, but the decades that followed have only revealed inadequate funding, overstretched social workers and a growing population of homeless folks who can neither afford medicine nor care for themselves.

As you'll see in the following stories, daily life at the South Carolina State Hospital wasn't always pleasant, but it did employ caring and empathetic professionals who were fully committed to making the hospital better.

1.

THE HOSPITAL HISTORIAN

You will find people who say they hated it and others who say they wished to hell they still had it, and they are both correct.
—Woody Harris

"A LITTLE MINI-CITY"

When I told Woody Harris of my plans to write a series of articles on the people who lived and worked at the South Carolina State Hospital, he warned me that their stories would be very different. "What you're going to find are people who will swear that [the hospital] was utter horror and that it was immoral," he said. "Then, you will have others that will tell you it was wonderful and that it was absolutely what they needed to stabilize them. You will find people who say they hated it and others who say they wished to hell they still had it, and they are both correct."

Perhaps no institution in recent history has polarized South Carolinians like the old hospital at 2100 Bull Street in Columbia. Opened in the 1820s as the South Carolina Lunatic Asylum, the Department of Mental Health (DMH) changed the facility's name to the South Carolina State Hospital for the Insane in 1896 and then to the South Carolina State Hospital the following century.[3] Harris arrived at Bull Street nearly forty years ago while completing a Ph.D. in counseling and adult education at the University of Georgia. "In the early 1970s, the 'feds' were jumping all over institutions, saying we needed to have a basic level of services for clients," said Harris, now sixty-four years old.[4] "They brought me in to establish an adult patient education program, both in academics and teaching 'living with illness' type skills."

But the job was hardly the educator's first experience working with the mentally ill. As a graduate student in Virginia, he took an internship at Eastern State Hospital in Williamsburg, the nation's oldest state psychiatric facility. "I thought it was the most interesting damn place I'd ever been to in my life," he said of Eastern State Hospital. "It was horrible in a lot of ways, and it was wonderful in a lot of ways. But you did stuff that was incredibly interesting, and

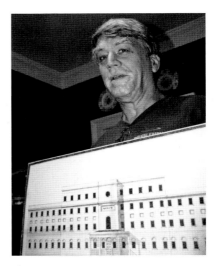

State Hospital historian and former employee Woody Harris. *Courtesy of author.*

you had a lot of diversity." Harris is one of the few people who can say he worked in both the oldest (Virginia) and second-oldest (South Carolina) state hospitals in the United States. The glaring difference between the two hospitals was that the Bull Street facility was massive. In the early 1960s, Bull Street held 6,600 patients.[5] In 1971, that total was down to around 3,000, when Harris, a Norfolk, Virginia native, took his post as the hospital's director of education.[6] His office was on the second floor of the Babcock building, a gargantuan 215,000-square-foot structure assembled according to the 1854 asylum model of psychiatrist Thomas Kirkbride.[7] Its design featured three wings branching out from either side of the administration building. Males were housed on the north side of the building, and females were on the south side, while the least functional patients were kept in the wards farthest from the center.

During his first twenty years at the hospital, Harris spent most of his days teaching patients skills such as reading, cooking and how to function with debilitating illnesses, including schizophrenia. In turn, Harris's patients taught him things like how to play chess and speak French. "You had to be kind of careful, because you could get very attached to patients you worked with for a long time," he explained. "There were patients that I considered my friends....We used to have a real mix of people; we'd get professional golfers, high school teachers, hobos and bums…all kinds of people all mixed in."

The former director said that, while the hospital had its share of incurable, regressive and violent patients (among them, serial killer Pee Wee Gaskins), most of those who were committed were eventually released. "People have the idea in this state, like most other states, that people went into the state hospital and never came out. That's not true," Harris said. "Yeah, they would go in there and they would spend a long time—six months, a year, something like that…but most of them got out." In fact, Harris claimed that many patients were stable enough to take off-campus field trips. "It's amazing to me how we used to take thousands of patients to the state fair and things like that, and [we] had very little trouble," he said.

The hospital also had its fair share of on-sight attractions and entertainment. Harris said it functioned almost like "a little mini-city," boasting its own theater, greenhouse, poolroom and gymnasium, as well as a canteen, church and ice cream parlor. On a large pastoral field in the middle of the campus called Fellowship Park, a traveling circus would even set up camp each year, fully equipped with tents, clowns and elephants.

"A FUNDAMENTAL FLAW"

While Harris admitted there were "episodic incidents" of patients attacking and injuring staff, he said he found that the community's collective fear of mental patients was mostly unjustified. Though there were several suicides during his tenure at Bull Street, Harris said he couldn't recall one homicide that occurred on facility grounds. Still, when he invited people to visit the campus, he said they would either decline outright or appear "very ill at ease" while there. "A lot of people think of mental patients as dangerous and all that," he explained. "Well, they are dangerous, all right. They're dangerous to themselves. They'll walk around in dangerous neighborhoods or on busy streets, and usually, they're the ones who get robbed and raped and attacked." Gravely ill patients were placed in high-security wards and rooms for this reason, while those prone to self-injury (Harris claimed several patients pulled their own eyes out) often had to be restrained and placed on twenty-four-hour watch. Obviously, the job wasn't for everyone, and there were times that the state hospital struggled to find nurses and orderlies to fill positions. Incidents of staff members assaulting and stealing from patients were not unheard of, and Harris said the administration fired several workers who simply didn't have the empathy to provide decent care.

While the hospital's forensics building (for mentally ill prisoners) was manned wall to wall with trained police officers, the other wards relied on civilian staff to keep things in order. One of the skills Harris's department taught DMH workers was how to decompress agitated, overstressed patients. He said attempts to calm patients frequently failed, however, because the asylum structure itself was so inherently stressful. He explained:

> See, you've got a fundamental flaw anyway when you put people in a psychiatric hospital. What society is saying to you is, "You're so screwed up and unable to deal with society that we're going to put you in a ward with thirty-five of the strangest and most difficult people from all over the state."…It was kind of fundamentally flawed, taking people who are having a great deal of difficulty coping and then expecting them to cope.

Despite the hospital's peculiar treatment design and diverse assortment of mental infirmity, Harris said many patients did in fact improve during their institutionalization. The most significant challenge, he asserted, usually came when it was time to release the patients back into society. "Basically, it's hard as hell to put them anywhere," he said. "Some counties don't have one psychiatric facility. As a result, large numbers of long-term psych patients who used to live all over the state ended up back here in Columbia, because that's where the best services were likely to be."

The DMH never had the funds or resources to establish an adequate network of services throughout the state. Hoping it would facilitate the reintegration of patients back into their communities, the hospital began placing patients from the same regions and counties in the same wards. But like so many strategies the administration conceived, this so-called catchment system was good for some but not all. While most patients improved during their time at Bull Street, Harris also witnessed many deteriorate.

> A lot of them would remarkably improve, but there are also people that we did a great disservice by putting them in [the state hospital].…The worst thing about working there, I think, probably was the fact that there were patients that it did damage to, because it didn't meet their needs and was kind of contrary to what they needed. There were people [there] that needed to be in the community with structure, and we didn't have it. It was cruel to them.

3.
HER SUMMER OF DISCONTENT

I didn't see any therapy. I didn't see any hope. It was helpless. What's so hard to understand is that there was no care for them.
—Linda McLamb

Nineteen sixty-one was not a good year to work at the South Carolina State Hospital. For the first time in the institution's history, the patient population eclipsed 6,600, well above its listed capacity of 4,823. The hospital maintained this population despite having an operating budget that ranked forty-fifth out of the forty-eight states with similar large public hospitals.[12] Without adequate funds for staff, facilities or treatment, hospital conditions were crumbling faster than Kennedy's contemporary Bay of Pigs invasion.

It was a shocking and hopeless scene that awaited twenty-year-old nursing student Linda McLamb (who, at the time, went by her maiden name, Linda Cox) when she arrived at the gates of Bull Street that summer. Enrolled at nearby Baptist Hospital's school of nursing, McLamb was forced into a unique rite of passage that every senior nursing student studying in Columbia had to go through—a mandatory summer of work at the state hospital. To make matters worse, she was placed in the Saunders building, one of four of the hospital's identical maximum-security structures that was built on the back side of the Bull Street property in 1955.[13] McLamb said Saunders was split into four wards: A, B, C and D, with A being the least dangerous and D being the most. Saunders housed only female patients, many of whom

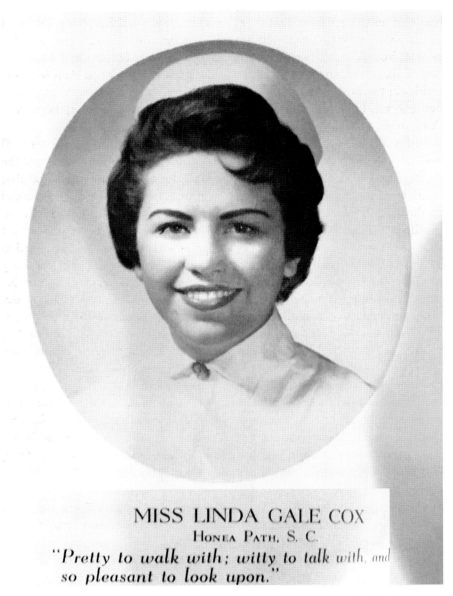

MISS LINDA GALE COX
HONEA PATH, S. C.
"Pretty to walk with; witty to talk with, and so pleasant to look upon."

Linda McLamb (a student nurse who worked summer rotation at South Carolina State Hospital) in the early 1960s. *Courtesy of Linda McLamb.*

had committed murders and other violent crimes but had been declared mentally unfit for the state's criminal justice system. "These were very sick people. You couldn't imagine them being in society or having a family or any of that," remembered McLamb, who grew up in Honea Path but now resides in Decatur, Georgia. "I worked on the C ward, and I can't imagine it being worse. It was unbelievable. When I told my family about it, they didn't think that a place like that could exist."

But it did exist, and it was where McLamb reported for duty, from 8:00 a.m. to 4:00 p.m., every weekday that summer. In those ninety days, the twenty-year-old South Carolina native saw a lot of pain and illness on that ward, but she saw little in the way of treatment from a trained, professional medical staff. "I saw the head nurse once in three months," McLamb recalled. "I didn't see one doctor or anyone trying to help [the patients]. I didn't see any therapy. I didn't see any hope. It was helpless. What's so hard to understand is that there was no care for them." Though over half a century has passed since the nurse's tour of duty at Bull Street, much of it remains seared onto her memory. Electroshock therapy (ECT) was popular at the time, and McLamb was often called on to hold patients down as they were jolted without the aid of analgesics or sedatives. "It was awful. I dreaded it, but we had to do it," she explained of the ECT. "These poor people, they could actually dislocate their arms and everything else. I'm sure they had a headache too, but no one gave them anything for it."

Incredibly, McLamb even claimed she witnessed the aftermath of a transorbital lobotomy on one poor patient. The woman, a schizophrenic, found a frog in the courtyard one day during recreation and hid it inside her body cavity, where it later died. When staff discovered what she had done, McLamb said, the irreversible brain operation was ordered.

> *I'll never forget it. When I came back to the hospital on Monday, she had two black eyes. She had had a lobotomy—that's the reason she had two black eyes. They let her on A ward after that, because she was like a zombie. The procedure made it easier for them to control her. I never did hear much about her after that. I guess that was the straw that broke the camel's back—that frog.*

McLamb's recollections from Bull Street paint a portrait pulsating with horror and sadness. In her memories, C ward was a hellish place where chain-link fencing stretched from floor to ceiling to protect staff members from patients—a neverland where patients' sobs mixed with the jangling of keys and the clanging of doors to create a bleak soundtrack. "I didn't see any improvement," McLamb explained. "There was no hope. None of [the patients] said anything about going home. It's almost like they were the forgotten."

At the South Carolina State Hospital, dances were occasionally held for male patients, where the nursing students were required to dance with them. However, at the time, there was no such social event in place for the female patients. With no television, music or any other form of entertainment to distract the women from their misery, the compassionate McLamb did her best to lift the patients' spirits, rolling cigarettes for them and playing cards with those who were mentally capable.

AN UNFORGETTABLE PATIENT

Although nursing students were warned to avoid emotional involvement with patients, McLamb became fixated on a gorgeous twenty-seven-year-old blond woman whom I will call Madison. "She could con the birds out of the trees, and if [staff members] gave her an inch, she took a lot of miles," McLamb recalled. "She could kill her own mother, from what we were told, and have no regret. I've forgotten a lot over all these years, but I haven't forgotten her. I was fascinated by her." An unabashed bisexual and diagnosed sociopath, Madison had earned a reputation as one of C ward's most explosive residents. "Even the other patients—as sick as some of them were—they knew not to mess with her," McLamb explained. "She had one way, and it was her way."

Seemingly everything about the twenty-seven-year-old beauty was deviant. Her boyfriend was serving a long sentence in state prison for murdering a woman, McLamb believed. Madison would write to him constantly and try to persuade McLamb to sneak the letters out to the mail so other staff members wouldn't have a chance to inspect them. Her convict boyfriend may have held a special place in Madison's heart, but he wasn't the only object of her affection. In fact, when she was allowed to attend a baseball game on the hospital grounds, she snuck off with another patient and ended up pregnant.

Soon thereafter, she escaped the hospital and was walking around downtown Columbia when police spotted her. Feeling she'd rather die than return to the campus, Madison grabbed a blade from her pocket and slashed her own neck, barely missing her carotid artery. She was rushed to the emergency room, stitched up and promptly returned to the custody of the state hospital. When McLamb met Madison for the first time several days after the incident, she still had a bandage on her neck. In quick order, Madison opened up to the pretty, brunette nursing student, telling her about her boyfriend and asking McLamb intimate questions about her own life and relationships that she didn't care to answer. "I guess she just wanted a buddy," McLamb said. "She just liked me. At the time, I was kind of attractive and she was attracted to me."

The young patient so enjoyed McLamb's company that when doctors tried to move her, she revolted in dramatic fashion. "They thought she was doing better a few weeks after the [neck slashing] incident, so they were going to put her on B ward," recounted the retired nurse. "That should have been good news, because she would have had more freedom, but that's not what she wanted." Fearing separation from her new best friend, Madison pulled off her bandages and ripped her neck wound wide open, splitting the stitches and pouring her blood onto the floor. Again, she was rushed to the hospital, where the injury was treated and sutured. When McLamb returned to Bull Street the following morning, Madison was back on C ward, sitting in a tub of ice water (an archaic hydrotherapy treatment intended to cool a patient's temper). "She didn't deserve that. That's for sure," McLamb said. "I just couldn't imagine how horrible that would be. But she was back on C ward, just happy as a lark sitting in that ice."

On her last day at the hospital, McLamb decided not to visit Madison, fearing a formal farewell might trigger an angry response from the mercurial patient. McLamb often wondered what became of both Madison and her child, but she followed her supervisor's advice not to visit once her summer residency at Bull Street was over. McLamb said Madison was between three and four months pregnant and was just starting to show when her summer term was complete. "I guess I was ready to move on, because I was probably getting too attached to some of them," she said of her patients there. "I saw what my roommate went through, and it was just hard for her." The roommate to whom McLamb referred was a fellow nursing student who suffered a nervous breakdown due to the trauma and neglect she witnessed while working in the hospital's geriatric building. That woman, who was just nineteen years old at the time, cried every day when she returned from the campus and eventually had to be hospitalized for her emotional state. After about a week of rest and treatment, however, she was able to return to the state hospital and complete her summer term there.

McLamb eventually graduated from Baptist Hospital's nursing program and returned to the Upstate, where she took a job in the psychiatric ward of Greenville's General Hospital. There, she helped doctors administer both insulin shock therapy and electroshock therapy, although those patients (unlike those at the state hospital) were given sedatives and Darvon to help them endure the physical toll of the treatment. McLamb later moved with her husband to Miami and worked as a nurse there until her retirement in 1993. She said that even though her stint at Bull Street continued to haunt her long after that summer of 1961, the experience proved to be immensely beneficial to her nursing career. "I'm so glad I had that experience, because when you're dealing with sick people, they're not themselves," she said. "So, I think psychiatric experience is a major thing to have when you're treating anyone that has had major surgery or a heart attack or something like that."

4.
A PASTOR TO THE PATIENTS[14]

These back wards were a ghastly systemic reminder of society's strong neglect of the severely mentally ill. They represented the bottom rung on a tall ladder of public disregard.
—*Tom Summers*

It's ironic that a man who spent forty-five years studying, practicing and teaching pastoral counseling learned one of his most important lessons from an old country bus driver. Yet, there was Thomas Summers in the summer of 1960, working in impoverished Williamsburg County at Trio Methodist College. As he darted from one of the three area churches to another, a bus driver, Rhoadus Blakely, called to him. "Preacher, come over here and hunker down with us. You look like you're too much in a hurry," he said. Summers went over to join the men, who were crouching down together outside of a church, killing time before they went in for worship. Reluctantly, Summers hunkered down among them as they watched the world go round and made small talk about baseball and the weather. In his nearly forty-year career as a pastoral counselor at the South Carolina State Hospital, this process of "hunkering down" would play a pivotal part in the way that Summers built relationships with colleagues, patients and students.

"SOCIETY'S STRONG NEGLECT"

Born seventy-eight years ago in Orangeburg, Summers was a terrific athlete with a passion for watching and documenting athletics. Even today, he writes sports stories and boasts enough college and high school sports memorabilia to dazzle an experienced collector. He went to Wofford College in the 1950s before attending Emory University's seminary, where he earned a master of divinity degree. He paid off his ROTC tab with six months of active duty in the army and returned to receive a parish appointment in Williamsburg. It was during this time that Summers got his first look inside the foreboding walls of Bull Street. He was accepted into South Carolina State Hospital's Clinical Pastoral Education (CPE) program and began working under Obert Simpson. Simpson had come to Bull Street in the 1930s and, a few decades later, remained one of only a handful of CPE supervisors in the entire Southeast.

Summers's mentor threw him right into the fire, assigning him to the hospital's back wards, where chronically ill patients would be warehoused for years, often until they died. In his 2000 book *Hunkering Down: My Story in Four Decades of Clinical Pastoral Education*, he describes his first impression of the place:

> *Nowhere were the excruciating ravages of severe mental illness so apparent than in the areas known as the "back wards." At this time, almost every public mental hospital in the nation contained similar tombs of hell. These back wards were a ghastly systemic reminder of society's strong neglect of the severely mentally ill. They represented the bottom rung on a tall ladder of public disregard.*[15]

As if this awakening wasn't rude enough, the first patient Summers tried to approach was a woman who cursed him before spitting in his face. "I never had felt so naked and stripped bare of reasoned thought in all of my life," he recalled of that incident. "She had gone straight to the heart of a foremost issue in my overall personal and pastoral quest—that of dealing with someone's anger."[16]

DELUSIONS AND ANCHORS

After completing his CPE training in Columbia, Summers's next stop was Central State Hospital in Milledgeville, Georgia. When he arrived there as a pastoral counselor, Central was already one of the largest psychiatric hospitals in America, holding over 12,000 patients (in comparison, Bull

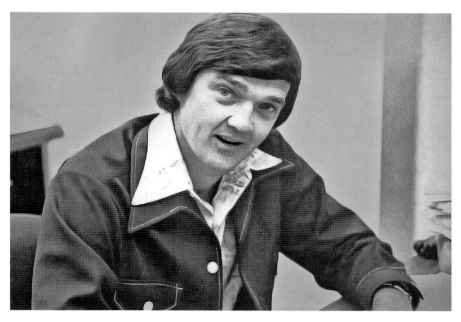

South Carolina State Hospital pastor Tom Summers in the 1970s. *Courtesy of Tom Summers.*

Street held about 3,500). At that time, ECT was extremely popular for treating depressed patients. Summers remembers spending many days in Milledgeville talking with patients who were waiting in line to receive ECT. The retired minister described his position in this setting as that of "a walking Rorschach card"; patients, doctors and nurses all viewed him through the lens of their own prior religious experiences and beliefs. This meant that some of them thought he was there to condemn, while others felt he was there to console and redeem. Almost everyone feared that he would judge them and governed conversations within his earshot accordingly.

Summers said that encounters with patients suffering from religious obsessions and delusions were commonplace. In Milledgeville, he met a man who had killed his young son because he thought God had told him to—just like the Old Testament story of Abraham and Isaac. At both Central State and Bull Street, he said it was not unusual to find patients who had removed one or both of their eyes, because they had taken the verse "If thy eye offends thee, pluck it out" literally. According to the retired pastoral counselor, a lot of mentally ill people obsess over and identify with a certain biblical phrase or character because they "give them an anchor," and provide a semblance of order and purpose in a world that they perceive as scary and chaotic. Summers says his mission was to lead patients gradually to the belief that God was there to help them, not punish them. But he says it was long and difficult work. "I think to take away any religious belief to which somebody is anchored, to try to remove that [belief] introspectively by getting them to think that through, unless they're ready to…can be quite damaging," he explained. Thus, "hunkering down" with the patients to earn their trust and attention proved critical to Summers's pastoral success.

"NO EASY ANSWERS"

By 1966, Tom Summers had taken over South Carolina State Hospital's Clinical Pastoral Education (CPE) program. By that time, Summers's mentor, Obert Kempson, had left the campus to work as a consultant with the South Carolina Department of Mental Health's (SCDMH) community division. Summers knew he had big shoes to fill. In 1967, he moved his office into the William S. Hall Psychiatric Institute, a newly built state-of-the-art facility on the Bull Street grounds that would soon become one of nation's leading psychiatric teaching hospitals. Yet, even with his recent promotion and the educational breakthroughs surrounding him, the Orangeburg native continued to take an old-fashioned approach when it came to counseling. As he'd learned early on in his career, there was simply no substitute for "hunkering down" with patients. In his book, Summers recalls teaching this lesson to a cocky young CPE student.

> [He] *had not yet taken the time to know the staff members as persons. Instead, he wanted automatic acceptance because he felt that ministerial prerogative deserved as such. I encouraged him to go back to his assigned ward and start hunkering down attitudinally with those in his surroundings or else he never would be soundly accepted as their clinical pastor.*

Though naturally patient, compassionate and intuitive when it came to relating to others, Summers was certainly not immune to the dispiriting nature of his work. On many occasions, especially in his earlier pastoral experience, Summers felt his faith wavering. "To me, there are no easy answers at all, in my estimation, as to why some people go through a mental illness and others don't," he explained. "I think being with deeply, deeply

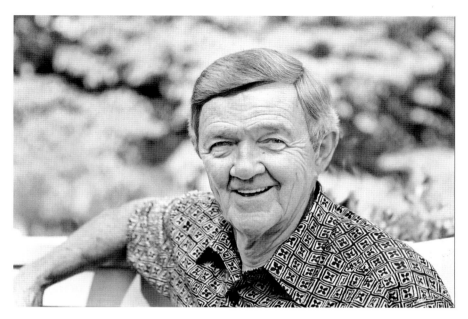

Summers in 2013. *Courtesy of author.*

troubled people like the mentally ill makes you question your faith. I started questioning my faith early in my seminary experience."

Ultimately, however, Summers said his experiences on Bull Street worked more to "embolden" his faith than to break it, claiming the patients he worked with consistently showed courage and provided a sense of hope. "I looked at it as being kind of a magnification of what [healthy] people naturally feel," he said of his interactions on the wards. "Life sometimes is tough, and life is filled sometimes with joy and happiness. The mental illness just magnified emotions that we all just naturally feel sometimes."

FROM BACK WARDS TO BACK ALLEYS

The early 1980s were a particularly tumultuous time for state mental hospitals, as DMH budgets shrank and the deinstitutionalization movement gained steam. Summers watched helplessly as his CPE department in the Hall Institute was reduced to half its original size. Patients spilled out of Bull Street and into the community-based treatment centers and halfway houses. Summers had to send his students and staff out to work with them. Of course, it didn't take long for deinstitutionalization's flaw to become apparent—it couldn't keep the mentally ill population off the streets. "It was a good ideal idea, but the doors opened, and you had a community out there that was not prepared," Summers recalled. "It often was said that many of the discharged patients were going from 'back wards to back alleys.'"

The retired minister said that in 1982, the National Alliance for Mental Illness (NAMI) ranked South Carolina near the bottom of the list when it came to the delivery of community mental health care. He also claimed that roughly 30 percent of the state's homeless suffered from mental illness. The progression of time brought about new ways of doing things for Summers and his CPE cohorts, and in 1987, he helped create a coalition of advocates for the mentally ill. "Some of the family members and former patients from these groups became literally my new teachers in the area of the mental illnesses," he said. "The anguish in their personal stories aided, as never before, the horrible welter of social justice matters and public neglect that surrounded the area of mental illness."

Summers's relationships with mental health advocacy groups opened a new door, and he began doing a lot of what he called "social justice ministry." During the days of the Reagan administration, he went to the Savannah River Nuclear Site, as well as Cape Canaveral, to protest the funding and development of nuclear weapons programs. He also campaigned for racial equality and, more recently, gay rights. One of his most important achievements was the orchestration of the first annual Mental Illness Awareness Walk in Columbia in 1988. For seven years, he served as chairperson for that march, which attracted thousands of people annually from the Carolinas and Georgia. He also began focusing on the language used in the mental health discussion in America. For instance, he argued that negative (but culturally popular) words like *nut*, *psycho* and *lunatic* work to propel the stigmas that have hurt the mentally ill for centuries. "In this ridicule, [the stigmatized] are seen less as persons and more as despicable objects of derision," the minister says in his book.[17]

Summers's last decade at Bull Street was a bit of a mixed bag. On one hand, medical and scientific breakthroughs did wonders to help the mentally ill integrate more effectively into their communities. The 1990s became known as "the decade of the brain," and they yielded medications that could help mentally ill individuals function better than ever before. The minister credited DMH state commissioner Joe Bevilacqua for fostering alliances with mental health advocacy groups, which dramatically improved

South Carolina's level of community care during his term, from 1985 to 1995. Unfortunately, budget cuts continued to haunt the DMH long after Summers's 1998 retirement. He said the most difficult effect of the cuts was the slow dissolution of the DMH nonprofit network that he, Bevilacqua and so many others had worked so hard to build.

Summers has spent a great deal of his retirement writing. In 2000, Edisto Press published his instructional autobiography, *Hunkering Down: My Story in Four Decades of Clinical Pastoral Education*. Six years later, Edisto published his second book, *Want a Frog? Memories, Sports and Other South Carolina Tales* in 2006. Now seventy-eight years old, the Orangeburg native is currently working on his first novel, which is tentatively titled *Sabbath Road*.

5.
HORROR, HUMOR AND HEALING

It was bedlam. I tried to resign right from the start but changed my mind. I said,
"If I leave, I'm no better than anybody else." So, I stuck it out.
—Ruth Westbury

The first psych ward Ruth Westbury ever worked in was a Veteran's Administration hospital in Lyons, New Jersey. She had enrolled in a nurses' training program in Charlotte, and they'd sent her to the Garden State for three months of psychiatric training at the beginning of the 1950s. With the recent end of World War II and most advances in modern psychiatric medicine still to come, the experience was not pleasant for the twenty-year-old from Marlboro County, South Carolina. "At that time, there was no psychotropic medication or anything like that, and that's when I decided I'd never work in psychiatry," she explained.

Little did Westbury know that she would find her calling, fifteen years later, at the South Carolina State Hospital. First, though, she wanted to start a family. After completing her nurse's training, Westbury married her high school sweetheart, Hugh, whose job with the South Carolina Forestry Commission took the couple first to Orangeburg and then Columbia. Westbury spent the first dozen years of her marriage giving birth to and raising four children. When she decided to return to nursing in the mid-1960s, Westbury found that places were reluctant to hire her because she'd been out of practice so long. The South Carolina State Hospital, however,

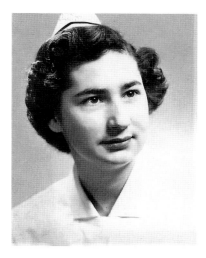

Former state hospital nurse Ruth Westbury in the early 1960s. *Courtesy of Ruth Westbury.*

had no such reservations. Westbury secured a job there and arrived at Bull Street on Valentine's Day 1966. It's hard to imagine a more tumultuous time to start, as the hospital was in the midst of its own racial integration. Each day, she said, there were roughly fifty new African American patients that arrived on campus, and like a lot of state hospital staff, Westbury immediately found herself overwhelmed.

"I found out that the patients coming in didn't want to be at the white hospital; they wanted to stay where they were (the all-black Palmetto State Hospital)," she recalled. "They were heavily medicated, and we had to screen them. It was bedlam. I tried to resign right from the start, but the supervisor left that night, and by the time she came back, I'd changed my mind. I said, 'If I leave, I'm no better than anybody else.' So, I stuck it out."

"MAN'S INHUMANITY TO MAN"

Though she started as a staff nurse, taking care of geriatric patients in the Gibbes building, Westbury was promoted to head nurse within six months. She was then reassigned to a female ward in Allan, a high-security building at the back of the state hospital's campus. With far more people than room, patients were forced to live in close quarters and sleep in crowded dormitories. "Every day, when I drove in, I would say to myself, 'Here I go again, seeing man's inhumanity to man,'" she recalled. "That's what it looked like to me. There was no privacy, and there just weren't enough people there to help them."

In such cramped quarters, physical altercations between patients were frequent, and nurses and staff occasionally found themselves in harm's way. Soon after Westbury's arrival at Bull Street, a patient threw a coffee mug at her and hit her on the head. During another incident, a patient slapped her when she forgot to get a doctor's order for the patient to use the phone. "The other employees were upset with me because I didn't put her (the patient) in seclusion for that," she explained. "But I just hugged her and told her I was sorry and that we would get it taken care of."

Though Westbury was able to avoid more dangerous attacks, not all nurses at the state hospital were so fortunate. She remembers a fellow head nurse who was assaulted and raped in her own office inside the Saunders building, another high-security structure beside Allan. "The guy who raped her had been a patient in Saunders at one point, but [he] wasn't when this [attack] happened apparently," Westbury explained. "He waited [for] her with a switchblade knife. It was a traumatic thing, but she was an amazing person. They took her to the hospital, but she came back to work two days later."

"THERE WERE A LOT OF THINGS THAT HAPPENED OUT THERE"

During her twenty-one years at Bull Street, Westbury witnessed her share of sadness and horror. About a year after she arrived, she said a female doctor committed suicide in the Cooper building after sewing a patient's lips together. "One of the patients, a young man, had cut himself, and they had taken him over to the emergency room (inside the Byrnes Building) to get stitches," she explained. "He was cursing the doctor, and I don't know what else…and she put some sutures in his lips. Of course, that incident got reported, and they found her [body] the next day. I was very upset, because I was the one that had sent the patient to Byrnes. I didn't know her (the doctor), but I was just really shocked."

Westbury remembers another disturbing incident that took place in the Preston building one night when aides restrained a mentally disabled woman and locked her inside a seclusion room. Though it was standard procedure to conduct frequent checks on secluded patients, the woman was left alone and died inside. According to the retired nurse, it was a death that easily could have been prevented. "She had been dead a long time when they found her," said Westbury. "Everybody knew that if anybody had really checked on her, they would have found her much earlier."

Research of newspaper archives reveals the patient in question was likely Annie Noakes, a "severely retarded thirty-five-year-old psychotic," who died on January 15, 1984. According to the *Aiken Standard* newspaper, Noakes died from an epileptic seizure after thirteen hours in a straitjacket. Her death occurred despite hospital rules that required patients be released from such suits every two hours for exercise. Three nurse's aides were charged with failing to follow hospital protocol, and Westbury was even called into court to testify about the tragedy.[18]

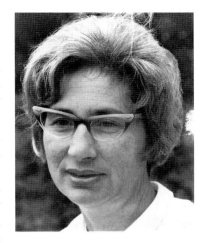

A young Ruth Westbury. *Courtesy of Ruth Westbury.*

Although the terrible incident garnered much-deserved media attention, Westbury claimed that incident was an exception rather than the standard when it came to bad things that happened at Bull Street. "There were a lot of things that happened out there that you wouldn't have heard about," she said. "There was enough bad press out there about the hospital anyway, so if anything could be kept out of the papers or quiet, they did it."

MOMENTS OF HUMOR

Despite the heavy emotional toll Bull Street took on its workers, it did, on occasion, offer moments of humor. Westbury claimed that, during a period of sustained negative publicity for the hospital, two state senators asked for permission to pose as patients and spend the night on the grounds. The hospital agreed, and they were placed in the high-security Preston building. When they arrived and asked to be shown to their rooms, staff informed them that new patients were required to sleep in the open dormitory with dozens of others. Terrified, they were able to convince two other patients, who did have private rooms, to let them sleep in their rooms for the night. They then asked staff members for the keys, so they could lock the rooms from the inside. When the staff members refused, the senators pushed their bedside tables up against the doors, so no one could come in. "We didn't hear too much from them after that," Westbury admitted. "It always amused me that they wanted to see what it would feel like to come in there as a patient, and when they did, they wanted no part of it."

Another morbidly amusing incident involved a catatonic patient who nurses were certain had died. According to Westbury, it was the nurses' duty to dress deceased patients and prepare them for the morgue (inside the Ensor building). When Westbury couldn't get the patient's blood pressure reading or detect any sign of respiration from her, Westbury was sure she'd passed away. "We even called a doctor, and he came to see her and said there was nothing he could do," she said. And yet, Westbury claimed, when staff arrived at the morgue with the patient, she suddenly regained consciousness, stirred to life and scared everyone to death. In no time at all, the patient was back in her ward as if nothing had even happened.

Westbury has other wild stories: she watched patients howl at windows while having LSD flashbacks, she saw notorious serial killer Pee Wee Gaskins in the Saunders building and she got to know an older patient who she claimed was one of the last to receive a lobotomy at the state hospital. Westbury also remembers a male patient who wrote a letter to President Lyndon Johnson that declared: "You need to come do something about this nurse, Ruth Westbury. She is too damn sexy for her own good."

"YOU HAVE TO LOVE THE PATIENTS"

There is one incident that Westbury uses to provide crucial insight into her Bull Street education. One day, just before Christmas, a female patient attempted to give her a bottle of lotion. When Westbury informed her that nurses couldn't take gifts from patients, the woman broke down, lamenting that no one at the hospital would accept her gesture of kindness. "I learned there's a two-way street, and while it might not be what you want, letting people give to you is something that can make them very happy," she said. "I learned that even though [the patients] had their problems, they wanted to do something for someone." Westbury claimed such lessons made her a better, more understanding wife, mother and daughter. "Working there taught me that mental illness was just as much an illness as any physical illness," she reflected. "You can give patients pills, and they might control the symptoms, but they won't cure it. You have to love the patients and let them be themselves and feel like they are needed somewhere."

By the time Westbury left the hospital, it had changed drastically from the chaotic institution she entered in the 1960s. The patient population

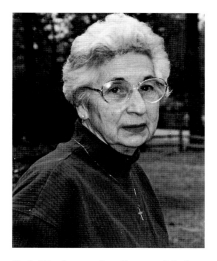

Ruth Westbury today. *Courtesy of Ruth Westbury.*

had fallen from nearly four thousand to under seven hundred, as medication improved and deinstitutionalization swept the country.[19] "From the time I started to the time I left, [the hospital] had changed from warehousing to treatment," she said. "When I left, it was a much better place, and I felt like I could finally leave it."

So, one day in 1988, Westbury finally said goodbye to Bull Street and all the dedicated professionals she'd come to know and love there. They held a reception in her honor and even named a conference room after her. Today, over three decades after she retired from nursing, a portrait of Westbury remains on display at G. Werber Bryan Psychiatric Hospital in Columbia. It hangs in fitting tribute to the woman who found her calling in the unlikeliest of places.

I didn't know what I was walking into when I applied at the state hospital. Every day was a new lesson in life. It was my calling, and I believe that firmly. I always said I wanted to be a pediatric nurse and that the last place I would work would be a psychiatric hospital, but I found out that psychiatric patients are a lot like children. They want to be understood, and they want to know what's going on. It was a good life experience, and I don't regret any part of it.

6.
THE HALL CHILDREN

I do remember this about my dad: he would go out of his way to speak to patients. He would take time off and talk with anybody that he passed in the hall on the way to his office. Even back then, I admired that about him. I thought that was unusual. Of all the things I took from my dad, that would probably be the number one thing.
—Carol Hall-Martin

I n its full history, which spanned two centuries, South Carolina State Hospital only produced one true icon: Dr. William S. Hall, who came to the institution as a psychiatrist in the 1930s. Hall became the hospital's superintendent the following decade and was named the state's first mental health commissioner in 1964.[20] Despite growing up in poverty in Wagener, South Carolina, Hall managed to become a doctor and put both his younger brothers through medical school. He was inducted into the South Carolina Hall of Fame in 1975 and is widely credited with bringing both the state hospital and the South Carolina Department of Mental Health (DMH) into the twentieth century.

Hall retired in 1983 and died in 1995; his longtime wife, Oxena, and eldest son, William Jr., have also since passed away, but his other two children remain very much alive and well. As both Richard Hall and Carol Hall-Martin tell it, their dad was a man who lived for his job. "He had no hobbies. He didn't play golf. There was no after-work interest

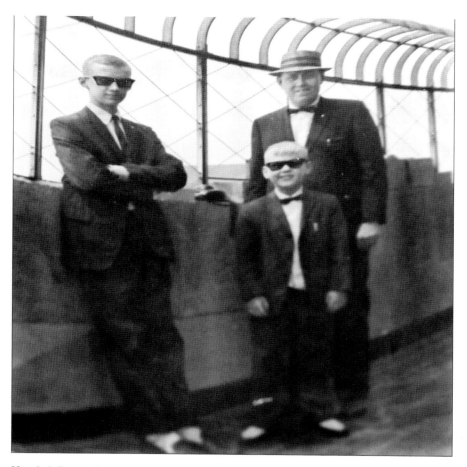

Hospital director William S. Hall and his two sons, William Jr. (*left*) and Richard (*right*). *Courtesy of Carol Hall Martin.*

that he had," remembers Carol, now sixty-eight years old and living in Chapin. "His first love was his job. I honestly believe that he cared that much about the mentally ill. He was always working. He worked on Saturdays, he worked on Sundays." Richard, who is sixty-six years old, validates his sister's claim. "When I was about to get married, I took my fiancé over [to the state hospital] to tell [my dad] I wanted to marry her, because I knew that was where he would be on a Sunday afternoon," he said with a giggle.

Hall was the superintendent of Bull Street when Carol and Richard were born. When they were very little, the family lived in one of the old doctor's houses on the hospital campus. They moved off campus in the mid-1950s, when the Department of Mental Health built the family a new home just up the road. While he was the superintendent of Bull Street, Hall and his family were treated like royalty in Columbia. The DMH not only paid for the family's house and a car but even supplied them with a gardener and babysitter. The babysitter, whom I will call Iva, was a patient at the state hospital, and Hall paid her to work so Oxena could run errands and have some time to herself. Both siblings have very fond memories of Iva, even if it wasn't always smooth sailing for the three of them. "I remember, one time, my mother was out shopping, and my sister and I were home," remembers Richard, who was just six or seven at the time. "There was a storm that came up, and next thing we knew, lightning hit the antenna going to the TVs. We had a pull-down attic, and when you just barely opened it, all you could see was flames." Iva rushed the children over to a neighboring doctor's house and phoned the fire department. The blaze damaged about a quarter of the attic and a small portion of the family's master bedroom, but the house was ultimately salvaged.

Carol recalled another day that proved traumatic for a different reason.

> *There is one incident that I still remember vividly. My brother and I were playing outside, and I had a toy gun in the holster. I walked into the kitchen, and [Iva] was in there ironing, and I said, "Iva, stick 'em up!" and pulled the toy gun out. And she said, "I'm a mental patient," and started crying. I apologized and ran outside, because I was embarrassed that I had hurt her feelings like that. I told my parents about it, because I was so worried about her. I was just scared that I'd done something bad, because she was almost hysterical.*

The children would often visit the campus on Bull Street when they rode with their mother to take Iva back after work. Both of them remember the grounds being well-kept and beautiful. "Every time we'd go over there, we'd see patients walking around outside, swinging on the swings or just sitting on the park benches," Carol recalled. "The groundskeeper back then did an awesome job. There were huge magnolia trees and azaleas as big as a house."

"HE KNEW EVERYBODY'S NAME"

Throughout their childhoods, Richard and Carol would continue to visit the hospital periodically. Every year, they would go trick-or-treating at the doctors' houses inside the Bull Street gates and attend a Halloween party for the patients in the hospital's auditorium. The siblings also took part in performances on the Bull Street grounds; the Halls were, after all, a musically inclined family. Oxena played piano at Park Street Baptist Church, where the family attended services every Sunday, and Hall served as deacon. Carol also played piano, while Richard chose drums as his instrument of choice. Richard played percussion in high school and later played in the University of South Carolina's marching band. When the William S. Hall Psychiatric Institute formally opened on the hospital's grounds in 1964, Richard played drums and Carol played ukulele at the ceremony. Richard even joined a band of seven patients who performed Friday nights in the hospital auditorium and occasionally played for cottages across the campus. A few years later, when Richard's varsity band at Columbia High School was preparing for a special performance at the Rose Bowl in Pasadena, the school asked Hall if

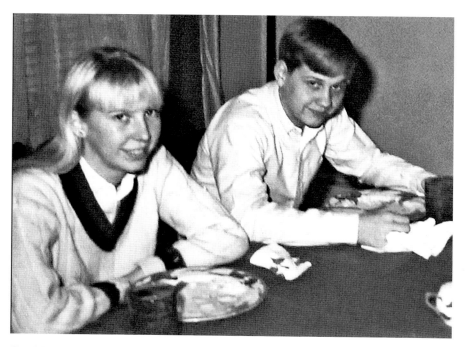

Carol Hall and Richard Hall as young adults. *Courtesy of Carol Hall Martin.*

they could use the hospital's campus to practice marching. Hall consented, and the school buses soon pulled up behind the Byrnes Medical Clinic, where the kids spilled out with their instruments.

Richard also got to entertain one of his other passions at the state hospital.

> *I was into electronics, and I liked to go over to the switchboard in the Babcock building and talk to the operators, and they'd let me answer the phone. To me, that was great, because I was just so into wiring and stuff. They would bend over backwards, because my dad was running the place. It was great to be able to do things that probably most kids weren't allowed to do.*

Richard was such an electronics whiz that he built a radio station inside the family's house when he was just twelve years old. A newspaper ran a photo of Richard at the controls of his homemade studio and his proud father standing beside him.

Dr. Hall's lofty standing in the capital city also proved beneficial to Carol. In the 1960s, the state hospital had its own off-campus dairy, where cows grazed. The man who oversaw the property worked at Bull Street, and Hall assigned him the task of finding a horse for Carol when she was in eighth grade. After the man found the horse, he kept the animal at his stable on the dairy grounds, where Carol would go to ride.

Along with Hall's status as one of the most revered men in the state, he was known for presiding over the hospital with infectious warmth and concrete humility.

> *I do remember this about my dad: he would go out of his way to speak to patients. He would take time off and talk with anybody that he passed in the hall on the way to his office. Even back then, I admired that about him. I thought that was unusual. Of all the things I took from my dad, that would probably be the number one thing.*

Richard recalled his dad fraternizing with hospital staff in the cafeteria.

> *Usually, someone in that kind of position isn't going to eat with the blue-collar workers, so to speak, but my father would go over there and eat at least a couple times a week….And the interesting thing about it is he could go in there, and he could tell you the name of the guy cooking his food. He was very friendly; he knew everybody's name and he made them feel like they were somebody.*

Hall's exceptional people skills and compassion for the mentally ill made him an easy choice to head South Carolina's Department of Mental Health. As DMH commissioner, Hall spent countless hours at the nearby statehouse trying to convince representatives to increase mental health spending. Once, he even bussed legislators over to the hospital to show them, in person, how bad things had gotten at the hospital due to a lack of funds. Despite having to work most of his tenure with a mental health budget consistently among America's lowest, Hall somehow managed to keep the hospital's doors open and accreditation intact. For the most part, the institution's conditions improved under his reign, as he worked steadfastly to put a major dent in an overcrowding trend that had started after World War II.

FINDING THEIR OWN PATH

Even after the Hall children enrolled at the University of South Carolina, they never strayed far from the sprawling campus at Bull Street. Richard spent his summers working at Dixie Electronics, right across the road from the hospital. Carol, meanwhile, went with a friend of hers, right after she graduated high school, to apply for a summer job at Bull Street. "I didn't tell my daddy I was going to apply for the job. I just went to the personnel department and filled out an application," she recalled. "I didn't want them to know I was his daughter and wanted to see if I could get it on my own."

That summer, Carol worked in the records department inside the Williams building, entering information into patients' charts. Stationed right next to the admissions office, she saw the despair of new patients on a daily basis. "You would see these patients, and they would be walking around so slow, dragging their feet. And I just felt so sorry for them…that they looked so depressed and down," she remembers. "I think people that know a mentally ill person look down on them. They don't think they are an equal, and I hate that, because mental illness can hit anybody and any family."

Unlike their father and two uncles, none of the Hall children chose to pursue medicine. Eventually, their lives took them toward horizons beyond 2100 Bull Street. William Jr. started college as a pre-med student but changed his major to history, which he taught for most of his life aboard naval ships. Carol, meanwhile, chose to go into business. She was part

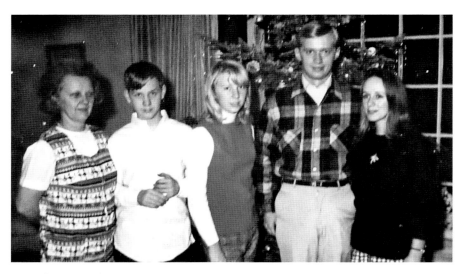

Hall's wife, Oxena, with their children Richard (*left*), Carol, William Jr. and his wife, Leslie. *Courtesy of Carol Hall Martin.*

owner of a crown and bridge dental lab until her retirement a decade ago. Richard continued to follow his passion for radio, which landed him a part-time gig at WNOK in Columbia. Soon, he would cross the bridge into television, becoming a news reporter and then a news director while he was still in his twenties. Over the years, he worked for television stations in Knoxville and Charlotte before returning to Columbia to end his career at WIS about a decade ago.

When Hall, the iconic DMH superintendent, finally retired in 1983, he and Oxena moved out of their state-provided home and into a house in Forest Acres, where Richard lives today. Retirement, of course, proved quite an adjustment to a workaholic like Hall, especially when it coincided with the death of his beloved poodle, Jacque. "When that dog died, he called me, and that is the one and only time I can ever remember hearing my daddy cry," said Carol. "I never saw him cry when his mother died or when his brothers died. When that dog died, he tried to give him mouth-to-mouth [resuscitation]. He loved that dog."

Following Jacque's death, Hall made it clear to the family that he did not want another dog, because the loss was so devastating. But Carol got him one anyway—a cocker spaniel he named "Cocky" after both the breed of the dog and his family's love for the Gamecocks.

He needed something that would take up his time and that he would have some kind of interest in, because he didn't play golf. He didn't do anything. So, I gave him that dog, and he pitched a fit, but that was the best thing I ever gave him. He walked that dog morning, noon and night despite the fact that they had a fenced-in backyard.

"ROLLING IN HIS GRAVE"

Mercifully, Cocky would outlive his owner, sparing him the heart-wrenching loss of another beloved dog. In the final years of his life, Hall suffered a stroke at his Forrest Acres home that left him paralyzed from the waist down. Requiring round-the-clock care, he moved into the Tucker Center, a nursing home right behind the state hospital property on Harden St. In a final salute to his many years of service, the Department of Mental Health picked up the bill for his care. "The DMH rolled out the red carpet and put him up for the rest of his life," explained Richard. "I'm surprised they did that for him, because they didn't have to. He liked it, because all of his friends would come by and see him. His mind never stopped working. That was the great thing."

On April 10, 1995, Dr. William Stone Hall's body finally gave up. He was buried at Southland Memorial Gardens in West Columbia. His wife, Oxena, joined him nearly nineteen months later. Both surviving Hall children are grateful their dad didn't live long enough to see the closing of the iconic hospital and the sale of its property. "I'm sure my father's rolling in his grave," lamented Richard. "They've torn down everything that he built up, in my opinion, by closing the Bull Street campus. These [mentally ill] people have nowhere to go. You go into an emergency room, and they're clogged up with people that need to be in a facility like that."

Richard believes the current mental health treatment model is so ineffective that states will eventually return to the psychiatric hospital model. "I'm not saying it needs to be as big or elaborate as it was, but they've got to do something. What they have now just is not working if you ask me," he said. Carol agreed. "I'm so glad my dad isn't here to see this," she said of the current redevelopment of Bull Street. "If it had to be something, I'm happy to see a ballpark there, but I don't like the idea of them trying to turn [the property] into a virtual town. Call me old fashioned, but that should be a place dedicated to the mentally ill."

7.
DESTINY ON A HIGH SCHOOL FIELD TRIP

It was just criminal to me, but when I demanded an autopsy, everybody laughed.
My supervisors were very sympathetic, but I remember one of them saying, "You
can't beat your head against the wall about all these incidents, or you won't be
able to work here. You just won't be able to stand it."
—Sue Cochran

In 1959, the Beatles, the draft and the civil rights movement still seemed a long way off. For many of the patients at the South Carolina State Hospital, hope seemed even more distant. Sue Cochran witnessed their misery firsthand when her Beaufort High School psychology class took a field trip to Columbia that year. Their first stop was a women's prison. The second was Bull Street. "I was mortified, because the prisoners had televisions, decent food and clothes, and everything was nice. Then, we went to the state hospital, and it was the total other end of the spectrum," Cochran recalled. "It was hideous, just barbaric. This was in 1959, and I just never got that out of my mind. It just struck me as the worst thing I've ever seen."

Newspaper archives from that year suggest that overcrowding and underfunding were to blame for the deplorable conditions Cochran observed. In 1959, the state hospital had 6,537 patients and spent an average of $2.37 on each of them daily, far below the national average of $3.61 per patient.[21] While hospital superintendent William S. Hall urged state legislators to increase funding to his institution, Cochran did her part to improve mental healthcare in the state. In the year that followed that life-changing field trip, she enrolled in nursing school in Charleston and began training to become a psychiatric nurse. As soon as she graduated, she went straight to Bull Street and applied for a nursing position there. "I told them I wanted their most regressed women, and I got more than I bargained for," she said.

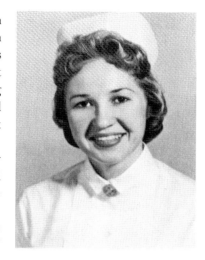

Cochran was assigned to the Talley building, which was built in 1904[22] and housed the hospital's most hopeless female cases. Many of the patients were catatonic. Their charts revealed they'd undergone lobotomies and multiple rounds of electroshock therapy. But what Cochran found most unsettling was how the women had ended up there in the first place. "The charts were interesting," she remembers.

Former South Carolina State Hospital nurse Sue Cochran. *Courtesy of Sue Cochran.*

"A lot of [patients] had been put there by their families, because they may have become pregnant or were dating somebody that their family didn't approve of, or they had seizures or something like that. It wasn't because they were mentally ill. They'd become mentally ill by being with all these other sick people [at state hospital]."

While the reasons they were sent to the hospital often remained unclear, the mental deterioration that had befallen them during their stay was glaring. The retired nurse remembers her first impression of the patients when she arrived in 1962. "They had to eat in their own cafeteria, because they couldn't leave the building," she said. "If a patient had on one of the state-issued dresses, they took it off before the day had gotten very far. Very few of them used the bathrooms. They had totally become like animals, and nobody cared."

Sadly, Cochran said "bath time" for the women consisted of aides herding them into showers and spraying them down with a hose. Though only twenty-one years old and brand new to the state hospital, Cochran refused to stand for such neglect. She instituted a toilet-training system in which she assigned each nurse's aide about a dozen patients. They were responsible for getting the patients to the bathroom and making sure they received a proper bath twice a week. Within six months, the Talley building's bathroom and bath policies had seen a complete overhaul. "It sounds like a silly thing, but it was a big deal, because we had to give them back their dignity somehow," said the retired nurse. "It still means a lot to me that I was able to do that,"

In 1964, Cochran's husband graduated from the Citadel, and she left the hospital for a couple years. When he flew out to Vietnam in 1966, however, she rushed back to Bull Street and requested a return to the Talley building. She missed the patients there; not only had she managed to memorize all 115 of their names, but she also actually took time each day to pray for every single one.

As the tumultuous 1960s brought change to America, the hospital continued to face the same overcrowding and understaffing problems that had plagued it since World War II. Cochran was the lone nurse in the Talley building, and with minimal assistance from doctors, she said it was up to her and the nurse's aides to take care of all the women there. And while some nurses at Bull Street struggled to get along with their aides, Cochran insisted she always performed the same unpleasant, physically demanding work that they did. Gradually, she earned their respect and maintained substantial influence over them, helping quiet their concerns when desegregation significantly altered the patient population in the mid-1960s.

Make no mistake, being a nurse at the state hospital was exhausting, gut-wrenching work, and Cochran encountered her fair share of institutional heartbreak. One of her patients, for instance, was transferred to a different hospital and threw herself down a laundry chute. Cochran said another died of a collapsed uterus when the staff at Byrnes Medical Center refused to treat her on account of her "bad behavior."

> *I sat in the stairwell and just cried and cried and cried. It just broke my heart, because it was a simple thing, and it could have been taken care of so easily, but they just wouldn't try. It was just criminal to me, but when I demanded an autopsy, everybody laughed. My supervisors were very sympathetic, but I remember one of them saying, "You can't beat your head against the wall about all these incidents, or you won't be able to work here. You just won't be able to stand it."*

Like many nurses who were employed at Bull Street, Cochran also suffered an attack at the hands of a patient. It happened on a Saturday afternoon while the only working nurse's aide was on a different floor. She said she was delivering a food tray to a large, middle-aged patient in a seclusion room when the woman became aggressive.

She attacked me, throwing me around that room by my hair. I was just helpless. I thought to myself, "I'm going to die." Thankfully, another patient ran upstairs and got the nursing assistant. She came down and saved me, and some of the patients joined in too. They always took care of me. The patients would always come to your aid. They were wonderful.

In 1967, Cochran took a trip to Hawaii, where her husband was stationed. She came back pregnant but continued to work at Bull Street for the next seven months. Finally, she took a break from psychiatric nursing in order to raise her two children. In the early 1980s, however, she returned to nursing at the nearby Bryan Psychiatric Hospital in Columbia, where she stayed for about a decade. She then went home to Charleston, where she spent the last twelve years of her career working in the psych ward of the veterans' hospital. Today, Cochran laments the state of our mental healthcare system. "We don't have any psych beds anywhere," she said. "If you're trying to get somebody committed, you're in trouble. We have very good psychiatrists, but as far as inpatient treatment goes, it's just not available."

Incredibly, the South Carolina Department of Mental Health now provides fewer than five hundred psychiatric beds for the entire state.[23] As a result, specially trained psychiatric nurses have become a rare breed in South Carolina. And while Cochran claimed she never wanted to do anything else, she'll be the first to admit that her career came with an emotional price. "I wouldn't trade anything for that experience. It was very meaningful," she said. "But I always cared much more than I needed to. It kind of cost me in a way. It takes a toll on you when you give that much for that long. Psych nursing is very taxing. It's difficult."

8.
THE PUBLIC SAFETY OFFICERS

There were some fun times. It was probably the most rewarding period of my law enforcement career. At some point, I worked [in] every building at the state hospital. It taught me how to talk to people and how to interact with the mentally ill.
—*Sam Alexander*

CLOCKING IN

When one thinks about all the people who worked at the state hospital, the officers who patrolled and protected it may not be the first to come to mind. But the fact is, few employees there had as difficult and demanding of a job as the public safety officers. "I don't know where in the world to start or how to start," said Phil Parker of his twenty-five years at Bull Street. Parker went to Columbia High School before enlisting in the air force in the late 1960s when his draft number came up. In the fall of 1973, he was hired by the South Carolina Department of Mental Health (DMH) as a security marshal. His annual salary was $6,000. "The public safety side of it was a little bit scary—a little bit intimidating—because all of the people that were around you were mentally ill and not in good contact with reality," he said. "And there were about 3,500 patients there. Every one of the buildings was jam-packed."

Over the two decades that followed, Parker climbed the ranks to become a sergeant and eventually an investigator. By 1997, he was director of security for the entire DMH. As a public safety officer, Parker spent most days restraining violent patients who refused to take their medication. "Most of the people, we would just talk to and they were okay. They'd take their [injection]. Others, you would have to restrain a little bit, and others, you had to do a whole lot more restraining, because they were just so mad or sick or whatever," said Parker. One middle-aged patient in the hospital's notorious Saunders building would attack the nurses and aides every time they entered the seclusion room to administer her medicine. "She never would give us any trouble, but if the staff tried to do it by themselves, she was going to hurt somebody," Parker recalled.

When a six-foot-two, 270-pound twenty-year-old named Sam Alexander came looking for work at the DMH in 1978, it was Parker who hired him. A fellow native of the capital city, Alexander had gone straight from high school to a career in law enforcement. He was a cop for the city of Columbia for two years before heading to the DMH for better pay. He spent nearly a decade working at the state hospital's northeast campus, a site about seven

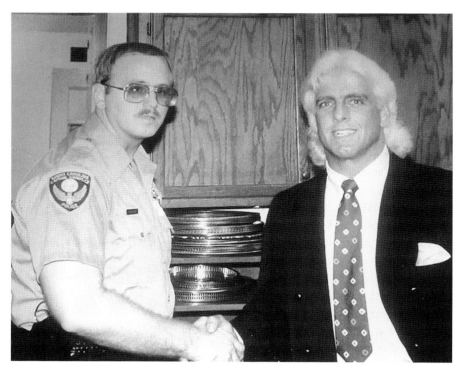

Sam Alexander (public safety officer at South Carolina State Hospital) and Ric Flair (*right*). *Courtesy of Sam Alexander.*

miles from Bull Street that included Crafts-Farrow Geriatric Hospital, Bryan Psychiatric Center and Morris Village, a state-funded substance abuse treatment facility. After a decade at the northeast campus, Alexander went to work for South Carolina Law Enforcement Division (SLED) for a few years. In the early 1990s, he returned to the DMH and was quickly promoted. "When I was promoted to sergeant, that's when I had to go downtown to Bull Street," said Alexander. "There were some fun times. It was probably the most rewarding period of my law enforcement career. At some point, I worked [in] every building at the state hospital. It taught me how to talk to people and how to interact with the mentally ill."

CONFLICT

As one might expect for two campuses that served thousands of patients, the South Carolina State Hospital saw its fair share of escapes. Most patients didn't get far. Usually, the institution's public safety officers would find them in a nearby neighborhood or bus station. Occasionally, they would even find them coming out of a liquor store. "Surprisingly, we had a lot that would drink on the run. They would actually be running and drinking at the same time," remembered Parker.

Of course, not every patient could be located or apprehended. Alexander remembers one patient in particular who fled from the northeast campus.

> Right after I came to work there, a patient took off, and I chased him into the woods, but he got ahead of me and disappeared, then went home and killed himself. I was sort of upset about that, because my partner didn't help me apprehend him. Sometimes, you'd have partners who were right there with you and then you'd have some that were just scared.

Parker certainly chased his fair share of escapees as well. Once, he even had to get stitches after a male patient swung a stick at him and sliced his hand open while on the run.

Even at his formidable weight, Alexander took his own share of lumps on the job. In one incident, an unruly patient broke his nose with a sucker punch. On another occasion, he found himself on the floor at the bottom of a dogpile of officers and patients. His back was so damaged by the weight of humanity that had squashed him, he was hospitalized and placed in

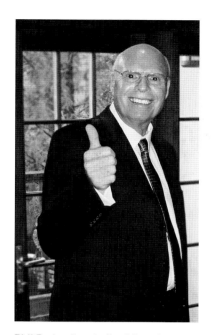

Phil Parker (head of public safety at South Carolina State Hospital). *Courtesy of Phil Parker.*

traction for a week and a half. Although he suffered no permanent damage, Alexander remembers one colleague who wasn't so lucky. The officer was working an incident in Hall Institute when he got a finger smashed in a seclusion room door and had to have it amputated.

Predictably, some wards and buildings were worse than others. As the designated forensics unit, the Cooper building had its own police officers and boasted the highest level of security at the state hospital. Alexander would often have to transport patients to and from Cooper wearing full arm and leg restraints. Other troublesome buildings included Preston, Allen and Saunders, which housed a lot of violent patients who had been deemed not guilty by reason of insanity (NGRI) by the court system. In those units, fights and thefts between patients were common. Parker said he occasionally had to use pepper spray to subdue and apprehend men who'd barricaded themselves inside certain rooms. Alexander, meanwhile, recalled some maximum-security patients who got so out of hand that every staff member on the ward locked themselves inside the nurses' station and had to hit an emergency button to alert the public safety officers.

The younger patients could also wreak havoc. "Blanding [building], before it was torn down, was not an easy place to work, because it had all different kinds of children mixed in there together," said Parker. "The mentally ill, the mentally retarded and autistic were all mixed together." According to Alexander, even the acclaimed William S. Hall Institute started to boil with unrest when it began taking in patients from the Department of Juvenile Justice (DJJ).

> *Somebody filed a lawsuit against the DJJ saying the inmates weren't getting mental health treatment, so the government told the director there to send their mentally ill patients to the state hospital, to Hall, so that they could get treatment. Well, if you're the commissioner of DJJ and they tell*

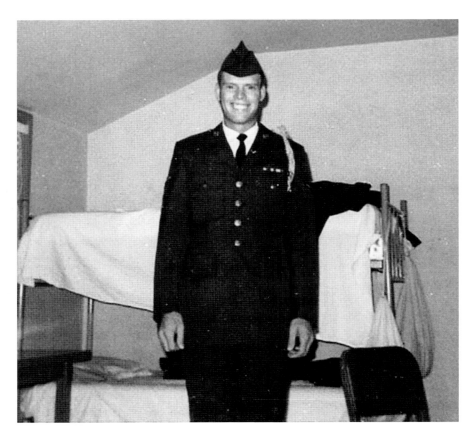

Phil Parker. *Courtesy of Phil Parker.*

you that, and you have these kids that are really bad, and that's the way you get rid of them, that's what you're going to do. You're going to say, "They're mentally ill," so you get them out.

Once these troubled teens moved to Hall Institute, mayhem followed.

They would riot and everything. They would tear the ward up. They would tear water fountains off the wall, commodes, anything they could destroy. They were real trouble, and they would escape regularly because Hall Institute wasn't made for those types of patients. They could throw a chair through a window and just get out.

CRIMES AND MISDEMEANORS

Though they had incidents with combative men, women and children, DMH officers generally found the state hospital's patient population courteous, friendly and well-behaved. "You started out kind of apprehensive, but once you got to know [the patients]…they'd be your friends and waive at you," remembers Parker. "My favorite part was all the different patients you'd get to know," added Alexander. "It taught me about the different types of mental illness. There [were] all types. I got to see some of them discharged and not come back. There were also some that died there and knew no other life but that, and that's sad."

Bull Street's public safety officers also had to respond to suicide attempts (both failed and successful) and transport bodies to the morgue. Another unpleasant (albeit less serious) part of the job was busting patients having sex on the property, usually in the woods behind the buildings. Sometimes, patients would even sell sexual favors just so they could purchase something at the canteen. "The oldest profession in the world went on at the state hospital with the patients," Alexander reflected. "They wore old house dresses back then, and some days, they'd have a whole dress full of change." Obviously, there was not much the officers could do if they stumbled upon such an illicit tryst. Alerting the nurse manager was usually the only form of reprimand at their disposal.

Though no employees were ever busted for that particular offense, some Bull Street staffers did manage to find their way into handcuffs. Occasionally, officers would arrest them for theft, threats and even domestic violence. "Sometimes, we would have disgruntled employees that would pull a fire alarm or threaten someone else that worked there," said Alexander. "I've even seen them come out there at night and pour a gallon of paint on their supervisor's car."

COMPASSION

With the new millennium approaching and the nationwide push toward deinstitutionalization gaining steam, Bull Street became a more pleasant place for patients and staff. "As time went along, there was better staffing, newer drugs, more activities," Parker recalled. "[The patients] got to go places around the city for different kinds of outings. It was easier for

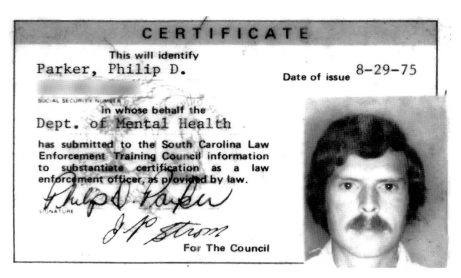

Phil Parker's work certificate. *Courtesy of Phil Parker.*

them to get privileges. There was also more freedom of movement and family would come and visit more." The retired public safety director said hospital staff would even take patients to fill out job applications so they could better reintegrate into the community. Toward the end of Parker's career at Bull Street, the DMH introduced a new course for its public safety officers called Prevention and Management of Aggressive Behavior (PMAB) and gave staff long-needed standards for handling patient interactions. Until that point, Parker said, most officer education occurred on the job instead of in a classroom. "Before PMAB started, you were kind of on your own—trying not to hurt, not to bruise, to do things as easy and humanely as you could."

Parker credits his parents for teaching him that sense of compassion. After two decades in the army, his father spent twenty more years working as a nurse at the Veterans Affairs hospital. Parker's sister was also a nurse, and his mother worked in the state hospital's laundry room—she was the one who first suggested Parker work for the state when he returned from the air force.

Alexander shared Parker's sensitivity to patients; one formerly combative woman took such a liking to him that she let him escort her to the hospital for her cancer treatments. He also did all he could for a proud war veteran who lived out his golden years on the campus.

He was an African American who had fought in World War II and had a combat infantry badge, which was very rare. I explained to my officers that he was a man's man and told them not to disrespect him. Every Veteran's Day, he would walk off from the state hospital. All he wanted to do was march in the parade. He earned the right to be in that parade, but they wouldn't let him march.

Parker and Alexander both wanted to extend their thanks to all public safety personnel, active and retired, for their dedication and commitment to SCDMH.

9.
TWO STINTS AT BULL STREET

I learned that some of the [employees] *at the state hospital had been there too long. They did not like to be corrected, and they did not like discipline. They did not like to do their jobs, and they didn't like people who insisted that they did them.*
—*Helen Skipper*

Helen Skipper is a rare breed of state hospital employee who worked two separate stints on Bull Street that were many years apart. Despite the decades stretched between Skipper's shifts, she experienced many of the same institutional problems in both. Regardless of her extraordinary work ethic and affection for her patients, Skipper's patience with her colleagues and the hospital's administration flamed out both times.

Skipper was born in Columbia in the mid-1940s and lived on Confederate Avenue, just a half mile from the Bull Street gates. Her grandmother Nancy was committed to the South Carolina State Hospital in 1926, soon after her husband died. "[Nancy's late husband's] relatives brought the sheriff and the welfare people to her house to try to take the children," Skipper explained. "Well, she cold-cocked the sheriff with a piece of stove wood. It was the 1920s, and she was uneducated with no real family, and they put her in the state hospital."

As a result of Nancy's commitment, Skipper's mother, Geneva, spent her childhood in an orphanage. When she became an adult, she went to work at Bull Street as a nursing assistant. It was shortly after taking the job that Geneva discovered Nancy was still a patient there. She asked a friend who worked in the administration department to check the patient registry, and sure enough, her mother was on it. When Nancy was finally released in the early 1950s, she moved into a small house and kept mostly to herself. By that point, Skipper suggested, her grandmother had become too "institutionalized" to enjoy much interaction with the family, though they did see her regularly.

Skipper's first experiences on Bull Street came early. As teens, she and her sister were allowed onto the locked wards of the Williams building to visit their mother at work. "I loved it. We didn't really see anybody who frightened us or anything that scared us, and the patients were extremely friendly to us," Skipper recalled. "They would come up and talk to us. Some liked my hair and wanted to touch it. That was OK with me."

FIRST TOUR OF DUTY

The year was 1964; the Beatles appeared on American television, Cassius Clay won the heavyweight title and the first Ford Mustangs rolled off the assembly line. After graduating from Columbia High School, Skipper took her first job at the state hospital as a nursing assistant. She was assigned to the Wilson building, a dreary old structure in which none of the patients could care for themselves. "We had [the patients] in cells, and we had them in beds with netting over the top so they couldn't crawl out," she said. "We had some who were catatonic and others who were violent. Some of the patients that we had in those units had had lobotomies in the past."

Skipper said hospital staffers were highly protective of patient records. "I'm one of those people that, if I'm taking care of somebody, I'd like to know what's wrong with them," she explained. "But if you asked a question there, you were pretty much told it was none of your damn business." As a result of that policy, any background information she acquired on patients was provided by her mother, who'd treated most of them over the course of her long career there.

While she said the Wilson building never seemed overcrowded, Skipper admitted it did appear understaffed. She said she never once saw a doctor working inside and claimed there were times that a single nurse was responsible for the entire building. Not surprisingly, treatment suffered. "We had patients over there that had bed sores down to the bone in multiple

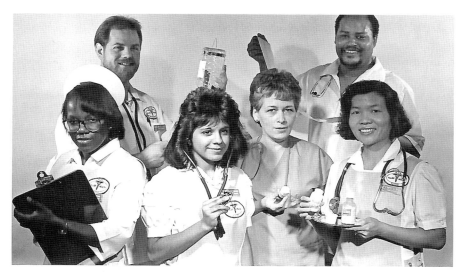

Helen Skinner (*second from the right*, former nurse at South Carolina State Hospital). *Courtesy of Helen Skinner.*

places on their bodies," she recalled. "There was no hope for most of them. They weren't going to live, but they could have used better medical care."

The staffing problems eventually took their toll on Skipper, who claimed she was assigned to care for three times as many patients as the other nursing aides. Eventually, she went to the hospital's head of nursing to demand an explanation for her unfair workload. When no satisfactory answer was provided, she quit on the spot. The head of nursing told Skipper that if she walked off, she would never again get a job at the state hospital. Fed up with an administration that was unwilling to help, the young woman walked away.

RETURN TO BULL STREET

After leaving Bull Street, Skipper earned her nursing degree and took a job at Baptist Hospital in downtown Columbia. For two decades, Skipper worked in Baptist Hospital's emergency room before becoming a travel nurse. When she finally grew weary of traveling, she returned to Columbia to contemplate her career move. While waiting for the answer to come, she decided to return to work at her old stomping grounds.

It was the late 1990s, well over three decades since she'd last clocked in at the state hospital, and the place had been mostly abandoned. The deinstitutionalization movement, which favored less-restrictive statewide community centers over a giant central state facility, had taken America by storm. As a result of this seismic shift, by the time Skipper had returned to work at Bull Street, less than half of the hospital's buildings remained in operation, and its patient population had declined from 3,250 in 1968 to under 350 in 1998.[24] This time around, Skipper was assigned to Byrnes Medical Center, a sprawling on-campus facility that treated state hospital patients suffering from physical illness or injury. She was stunned by the transformation the years had brought to the hospital.

> [The hospital] *wasn't anything like* [it was] *when I worked there the first time. Back then, you* [could] *go over to Byrnes and there* [would be] *surgery going on. They* [would be] *delivering babies, and there was real medical care. This time, it was pathetic. We'd have patients that you would have resuscitation orders for, but nobody over there knew how to do a code. They didn't know what intubation was. They weren't trained to do stuff like that.*

Skipper believes her fellow nurses at Byrnes genuinely cared for the patients, but because they'd been trained solely in psychiatric care, they were grossly incompetent when it came to handling critical situations. In contrast, her two decades inside Baptist Hospital's emergency room made her an expert in handling medically critical patients. As a result, she was soon promoted to the position of nurse supervisor in the Williams building, the same structure where her mother had worked four decades earlier. The experience was not a good one; from the outset, Skipper encountered resistance in her efforts to oversee staff. "I learned that some of the [employees] at the state hospital had been there too long. They did not like to be corrected, and they did not like discipline. They did not like to do their jobs, and they didn't like people who insisted that they did them," she explained.

Indeed, her opposition was fierce. During her second term at Bull Street, Skipper claimed fellow employees put sugar in her gas tank, poured acid onto her car and even sent her written death threats. She alleged that workplace tensions came to a head when a patient on Ward 121 sustained a broken nose and black eyes while in the care of three hospital staffers. The incident infuriated Skipper; she promptly wrote the women up and took the matter to DMH administration officials.

The last straw for Skipper came when a fellow nurse supervisor appealed to the administration, requesting that Skipper's allegations against the three women be dismissed. "I hit the ceiling and told them, 'Either I'm out of this unit, or I'm out of the whole system. I will not work where people cut my throat behind my back,'" she said. She was promptly transferred back to Byrnes Medical Center.

LIGHTER MOMENTS

Skipper's shifts at Byrnes were far less tumultuous than they'd been in Williams. She was no longer responsible for staff and could focus more on her patients. "I did love the patients out there," she said. "There was never one out there that I didn't like. I never had one that pushed my buttons the wrong way. I had some that were obnoxious. I had some that were sweet as they could be. Some of them had some really endearing qualities. It was hard not to like them." Her all-time favorite patient was an African American who was nicknamed "Gervais," because he often wandered off the Bull Street campus and up to the state house on Gervais Street. He called Skipper "Suzy" and was convinced she was his cousin despite the clear color divide between them. "He was just a very sweet man in his own little way," she said. "He always liked being brought back to the state hospital in a police car. He thought that was really cool."

Even Skipper's difficult 1964 stint on Bull Street was not entirely devoid of humor. Back then, after patients passed away, she had to transport their bodies to the hospital morgue inside the Ensor building. Though such trips were usually somber, because so many of the bodies went unclaimed, one particular trip proved quite comical. After one patient died at Byrnes Medical Center, Skipper and another nursing aid, whom we will call Everett, were ordered to transport his remains to the morgue. At first, Everett refused outright, terrified of getting that close to a dead person. At last, he conceded when Skipper assured him that he would not have to touch the body; she volunteered to ride in the back of the car with the body if he drove. "Well, we got up to the morgue and pulled the stretcher out," she recalled. "And when we popped the wheels up, the patient expelled air from his mouth, which happens sometimes. Anyway, they saw Everett running out [of] the Calhoun Street exit [of the hospital]. He was gone. It scared him to death, and he wasn't sticking around for an explanation."

ACTS OF COMPASSION

Any semblance of comic relief was welcome at Bull Street, as it was often a depressing and emotionally exhausting place to work. Even a seasoned nurse like Skipper, who'd watched hundreds of patients die inside the emergency room at Baptist, was shaken by a young AIDS patient who spent his final hours in her care. By the time the twenty-four-year-old arrived at Byrnes, he was bald, emaciated and suffering a fever of 105 degrees. For Skipper, the saddest part of this experience was how the young man didn't have any loved ones with him during his last moments. "My mother taught me that no one should die alone," she said. "So, when it was obvious that he was dying, I took off my gloves, held his hand and talked with him until he passed." After death mercifully came to the man, Skipper cried for her first and only time while working at Bull Street. She then dried her eyes, took a few deep breaths, put her gloves back on and returned to work on the ward.

In addition to the inherent emotional strains of the job at Bull Street, there were also a number of physical risks that the hospital's employees faced. Skipper's mother, Geneva, was forced into early retirement in 1981, when a patient attacked her in the Williams building. While Geneva and several other staffers were trying to push the man into a seclusion room, he managed to grab her and slam her headfirst into a wall. The assault permanently damaged Geneva's spine. Two decades later, Skipper would suffer her own attack while on the clock at the hospital. It was surprising, she said, because the patient was usually quite fond of her. "I turned my back on him, and what he saw was evidently not me but something else," she recalled. "He started beating me in the head, and the moment I turned around and faced him, he broke down and started crying." Except for a headache, Skipper was uninjured in the attack. And when other staff members urged her to lock the delusional patient in a seclusion room, she refused, choosing instead to go sit with him in his room until he calmed down. It was a signature act of compassion from the woman who'd first come to Bull Street as a teenager many years ago.

I see mental illness the same way I see physical illness. It is something that happens to us, and we cannot help [it]. *We just need to accept it, try to care for them and love them. We always want to label everybody, but I think if people actually worked around these patients and saw them as the humans they really are, they would feel differently.*

In 2002, Skipper left Bull Street to become a hospice nurse. Three years later, her mother, Geneva, died. Over the last decade, Skipper has retired from nursing and made a life for herself in the country, living on a large piece of farmland between Belton and Anderson.

10.
McMASTER BROUGHT PROGRESS AND CHANGE TO THE HOSPITAL

Most people think of the mentally ill as being defined by their diagnosis.
That's so not true. These guys had very strong individual personalities,
and I enjoyed being around them.
—John McMaster

For decades, John McMaster was a fixture at the South Carolina State Hospital. Inside the ever-changing mental health landscape known as Bull Street, he demonstrated extraordinary diversity over the years, serving as social worker, therapist, teacher and liaison. But no matter who his clients were, where his office was or what program he was spearheading, McMaster's commitment to the employees and patients of the state hospital was never short of commendable.

John McMaster, the older brother of the current governor of South Carolina, Henry McMaster, was born in 1946 in Columbia. As a teen, his parents sent him to Blue Ridge School for Boys in Virginia, and it was there that his interest in mental health was born. The pastor of the Episcopalian school had once worked in a state hospital, and his stories about the institution captivated his students. After enrolling at the University of South Carolina, McMaster studied psychology and earned a Bachelor of Science degree and master's degree in social work.

After earning a level V social work certification (the highest level attainable), McMaster headed to Bull Street to practice the things he'd learned, but the year was 1970, and the state hospital was severely crowded and understaffed.

McMaster became a clinical social worker at the hospital, but the high case load and endless paperwork made the job all but impossible. After nine months, he left Bull Street to work for the South Carolina Department of Corrections (DOC), where he said he and several others launched an inventive mental health program. While working in the notorious Central Correctional Institution (CCI), McMaster was eventually promoted to the position of director of social work services. "I was responsible for evaluating death row inmates, as well as any other inmate with mental health problems," he said. "I would refer psychotic inmates to the psychiatrist, who would prescribe psychotropic medication." His twelve years of intensive work with the DOC would prove invaluable when he returned to the state hospital a few years later.

THE NGRI UNIT

McMaster's second stint on Bull Street was vastly better than his first. He became the first clinical social worker to work in the hospital's new "Not Guilty by Reason of Insanity" (NGRI) unit. It housed patients who'd committed serious crimes but had been deemed psychologically unfit for trial. Instead of receiving a prison sentence, they were committed to the hospital for an indefinite amount of time, essentially until they could be declared mentally fit to return to society.

> *The NGRI program was way ahead of its time* [and] *probably the best in the country. We had total control of our patients, because they were under our jurisdiction. This gave us the opportunity and time* [we] *needed to work with the mental health centers…* [in order to] *better prepare the patient for re-entry into the community.*

To successfully return patients to society, McMaster and the other members of the NGRI treatment team installed a step program, which gradually advanced them toward freedom. For instance, a stabilized forensics patient would be granted a "yard card," which allowed them to roam the hospital campus freely for an hour. If they were well-behaved during this hour, they would be given another hour and another until they had full freedom to walk the campus whenever they wished. If no violations were noted, the patient would be transferred to a community mental health care program in

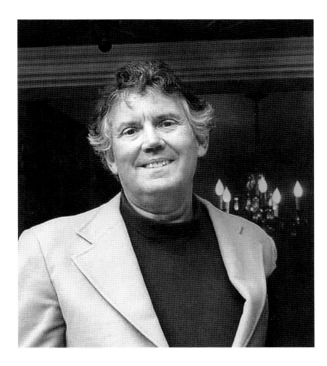

Former South Carolina State Hospital head of social work, John McMaster. *Courtesy of John McMaster.*

a different town. They would then be continually evaluated until they proved they could live on their own. Any missteps on the patient's part would result in them being returned to the state hospital.

The program proved to be highly effective. McMaster even recalled a former patient who went from living in a ward in the NGRI building to enrolling in his community's technical college. When the man's case manager asked him what had brought about his transformation, he answered, "If I don't do as I am told, John McMaster will haul me back there to the state hospital."

WORKING WITH STAFF

After working with the state hospital's forensics patients, McMaster was hired to oversee Bull Street's new Employee Assistance Program (EAP). "It was exactly what I had wanted to do all along," he said. "I had free reign to help the SCDMH (Department of Mental Health) employees and practice pure clinical social work." As the only licensed professional counselor and master social worker in the EAP, McMaster spent his last six years in social work helping state hospital staff cope with life both inside and outside the Bull Street gates. If an employee had a substance abuse problem, he would evaluate them and get them into inpatient treatment. If a staffer was having financial or personal problems, he would try his best to direct them toward the resources they needed. The retired master social worker even remembers one woman he tried to help out of a bad marriage.

> *One sad case was a young woman whose husband controlled her every move. He stalked her at work and wouldn't let her go out with friends. There are a number of well-documented warning signs, and her husband met them all. I tried my best to impart upon her that the odds were* [that] *he would eventually hurt her badly or kill her, but she refused to go to a shelter and never came back.*

Such cases took an emotional toll on McMaster, and he finally retired after working at the state hospital for a half dozen years.

> *While at EAP, I really felt for the overworked food service people and the young nurses. The community mental health counselors also had way too many patients. It started to wear on me, as I was the one therapist for the entire department. There were lots of sad cases, and my time was limited. After six years, retirement was a blessing.*

BULL STREET THEN AND NOW

Although McMaster retired from the Department of Mental Health in 2002, he remembers his old coworkers and patients with a genuine fondness. He worked hand-in-hand with the hospital's activity therapists, accompanying them and the patients to the zoo, fair and, occasionally, to Ryan's Steakhouse for lunch. These excursions enabled him to observe the patients in real-life situations. He would later share his evaluations with community mental health experts so that patients could be transitioned properly. McMaster's hands-on work with the state hospital's patients also taught him that there was a lot more to them than their illnesses. "Most people think of the mentally ill as being defined by their diagnosis," he explained. "That's so not true. These guys had very strong individual personalities, and I enjoyed being around them."

He also had only kind words to say about the nurses and aides who kept the hospital running, calling them "an absolute delight to work with."

> *People think that doctors were the primary change agents* [at the hospital], *which is far from the truth.* [The doctors] *had the least amount of contact with the patients; they prescribed medication and got feedback from the nurses. The nurses' aides were the most valuable people on the ward. They were angels and had, by far, the most contact and involvement with the patients. I liked them a lot and spent most of my time on the ward with them.*

Over the last decade, McMaster has been a vocal critic of Columbia's Bull Street Project, an endeavor to develop the former hospital campus into a mixed-use neighborhood. Despite the ambitious plans that were announced years ago by Columbia's city government, no apartments, hotels or movie theaters have opened there. Moreover, none of the hospital's major buildings (Babcock, Williams, Byrnes, et cetera) have been repurposed or razed—they continue to sit, rotting around the city's new minor-league baseball stadium. "The whole [project] was a lie, and the baseball park was more of an afterthought," McMaster said. "[You] think I might be angry about this thing? You're right. Who is going to come to Columbia to see this bottom-level baseball? It's mostly recycled money, with nothing much, if any, added to the economy." McMaster believes several of the old buildings should be renovated and restored to health. That way, they could serve not only as repurposed business establishments but as monuments to the patients and staff members that inhabited them for generations.

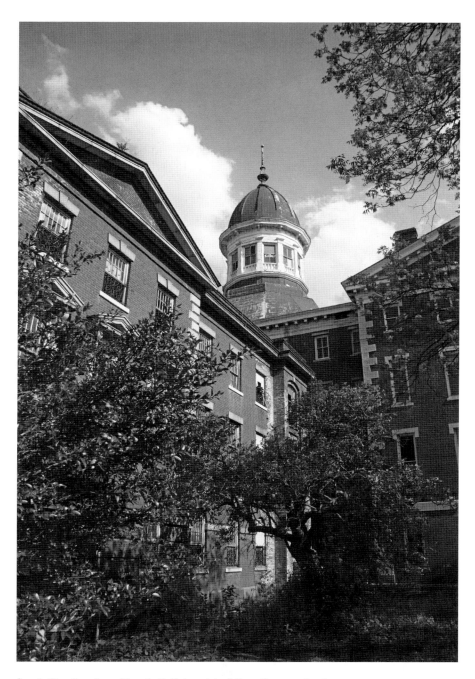

South Carolina State Hospital's Babcock building. *Courtesy of author.*

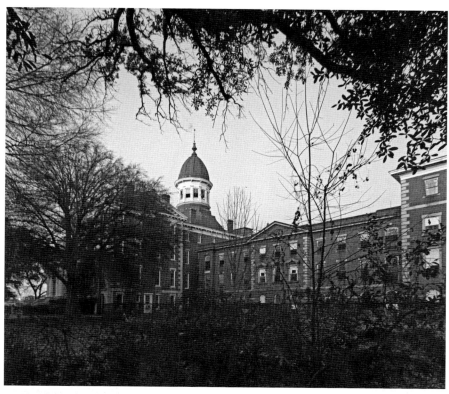

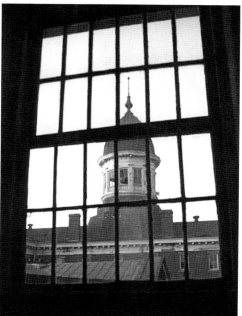

Above: South Carolina State Hospital's Babcock building. *Courtesy of author.*

Left: Babcock's iconic cupola as seen through a window in another wing. *Courtesy of author.*

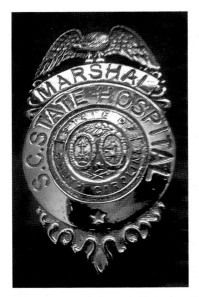
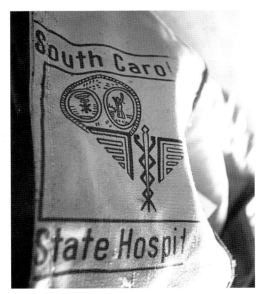

Left: State Hospital marshal's badge. *Courtesy of Sam Alexander.*

Right: South Carolina State Hospital emblem printed on patient coat. *Courtesy of author.*

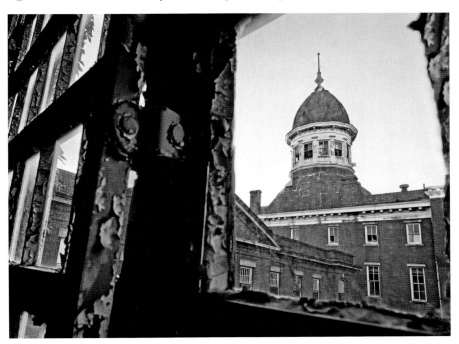

Babcock through window grill. *Courtesy of author.*

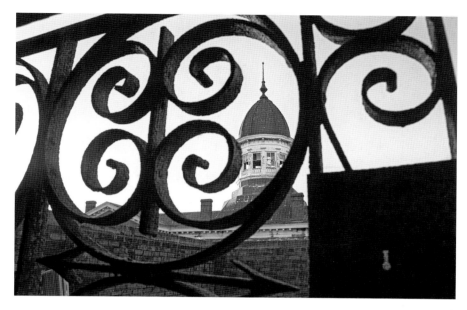

Babcock through locked window grill in high-security wing. *Courtesy of author.*

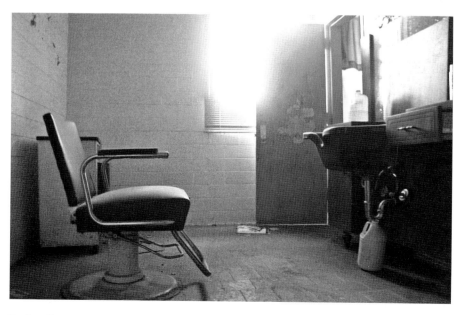

Barber Shop, secure ward. *Courtesy of author.*

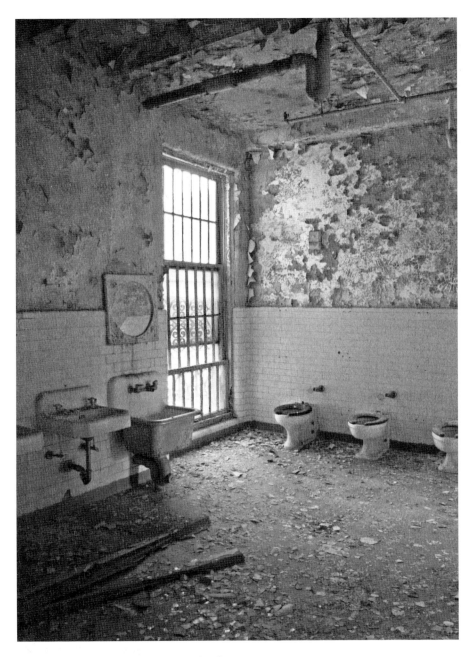

Patient bathroom, Babcock. *Courtesy of author.*

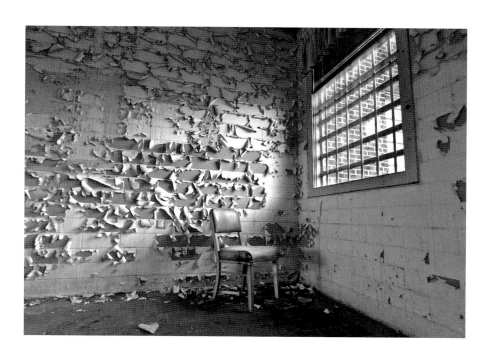

Chair and barred window in the forensics unit. *Courtesy of author.*

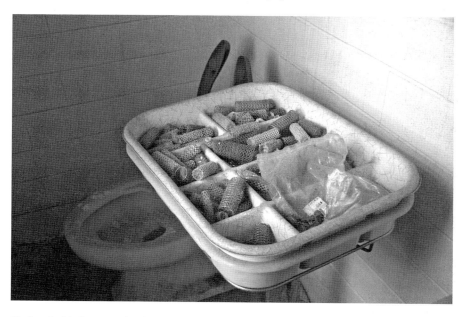

Curlers inside beauty salon in secure ward. *Courtesy of author.*

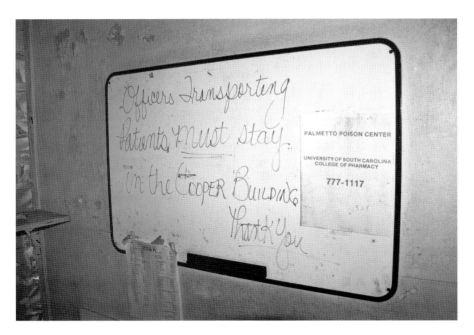

White board inside Cooper building. *Courtesy of author.*

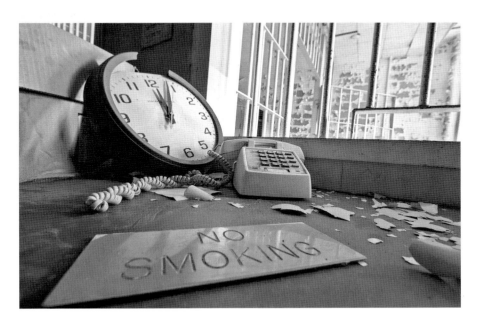

Officer's window in the forensics unit. *Courtesy of author.*

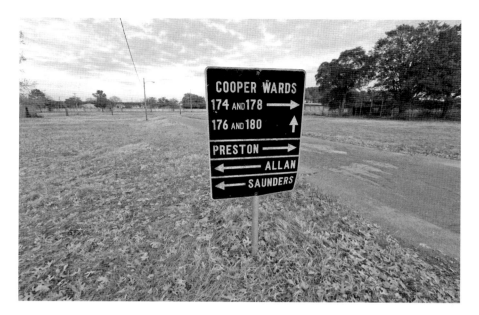

Sign for the hospital's back wards. *Courtesy of author.*

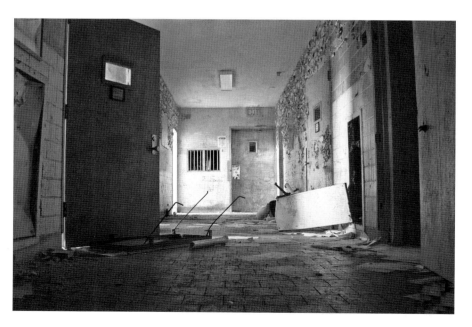

Ward hallway in forensics unit. *Courtesy of author.*

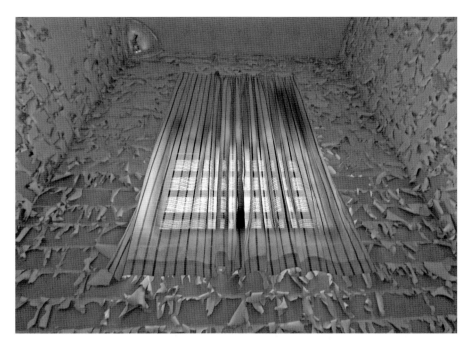

Curtains and window in patient room in secure ward. *Courtesy of author.*

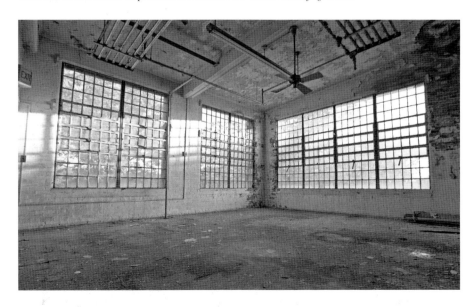

Sunroom, Babcock. *Courtesy of author.*

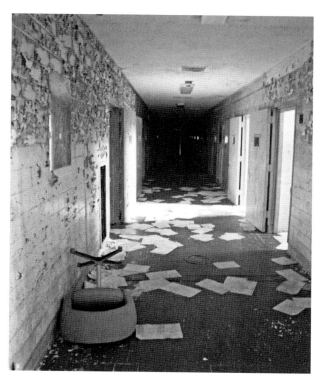

Left: Files on hallway floor in forensics unit. *Courtesy of author.*

Below: Sign for forensics unit. *Courtesy of author.*

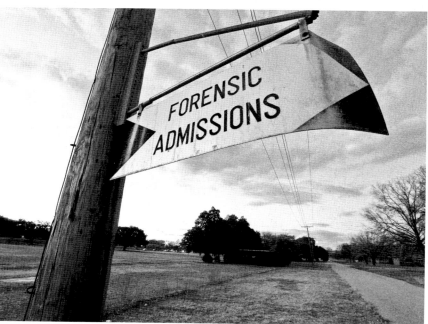

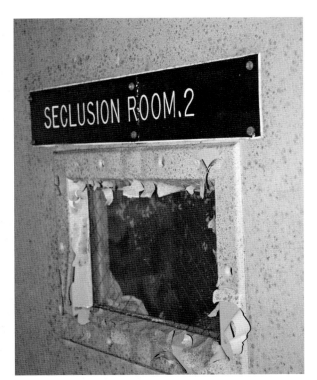

Right: Seclusion room in secure ward. *Courtesy of author.*

Below: Metal door to sunroom, Babcock. *Courtesy of author.*

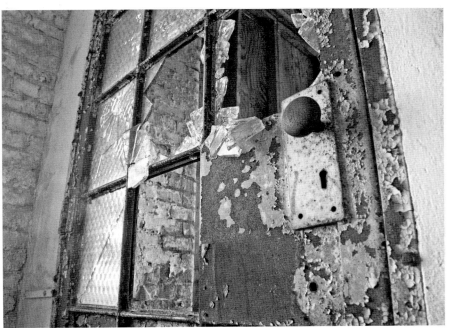

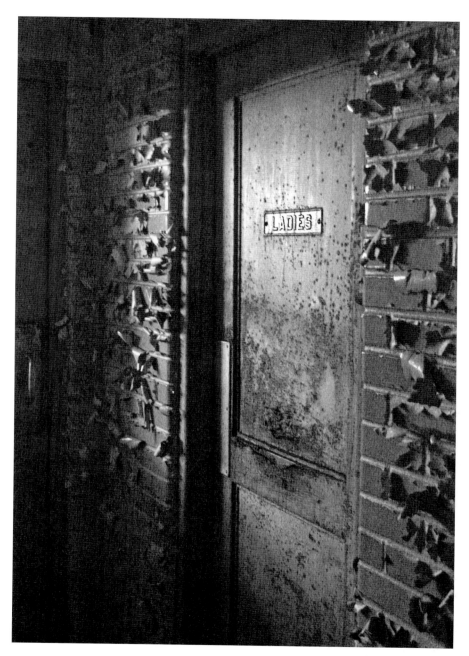

Ladies restroom, Babcock. *Courtesy of author.*

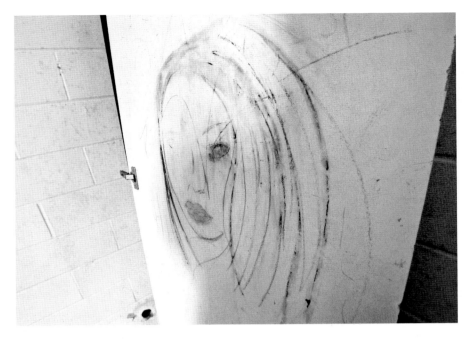

Sketch on a stall door in a bathroom in secure unit. *Courtesy of author.*

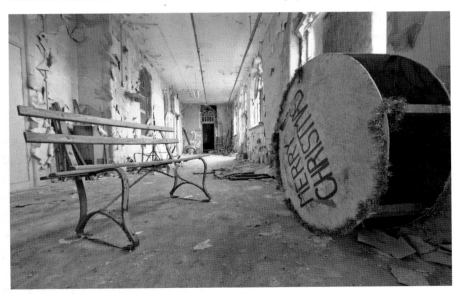

Porch, Babcock. *Courtesy of author.*

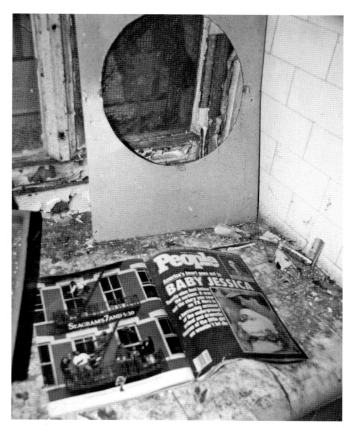

Left: 1987 *People Magazine*, Babcock. *Courtesy of author.*

Below: Medication room in secure ward. *Courtesy of author.*

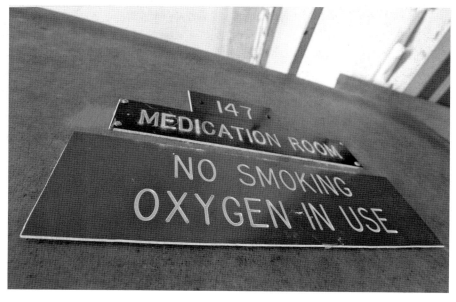

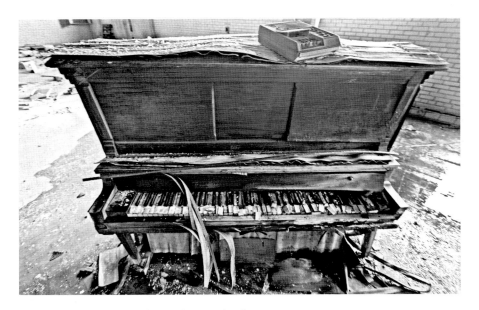

Piano inside hospital warehouse. *Courtesy of author.*

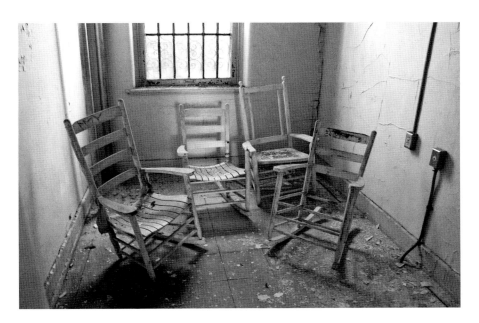

Rocking chairs, Babcock. *Courtesy of author.*

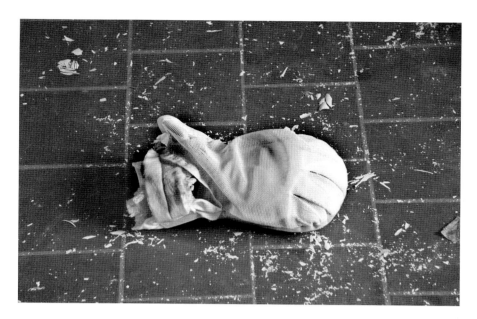

Restraint mitt in secure ward. *Courtesy of author.*

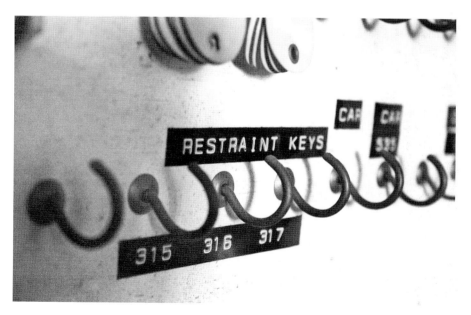

Key hooks in forensics unit. *Courtesy of author.*

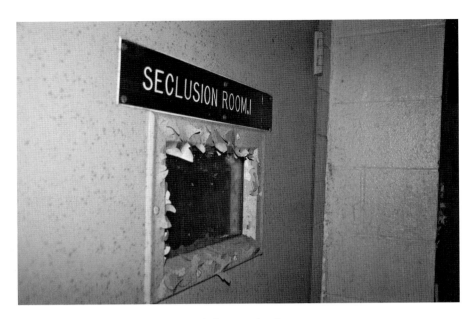

Seclusion room window in secure ward. *Courtesy of author.*

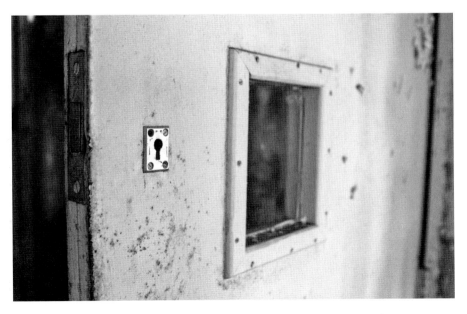

Viewing window of patient room in the secure ward, Babcock. *Courtesy of author.*

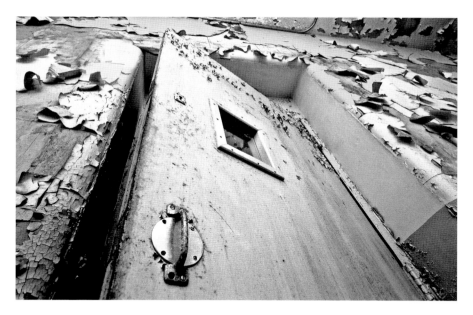

Door to patient room in secure ward of Babcock. *Courtesy of author.*

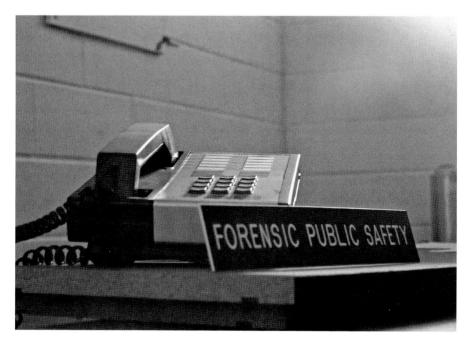

Telephone in the hospital public safety office. *Courtesy of author.*

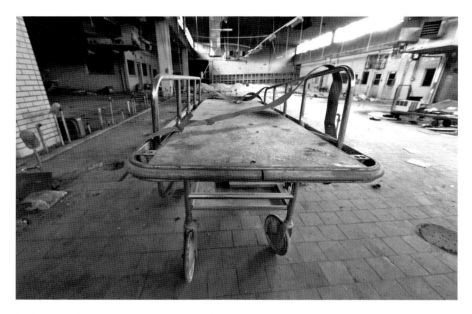

Patient stretcher in hospital warehouse. *Courtesy of author.*

Ward schedule, secure unit. *Courtesy of author.*

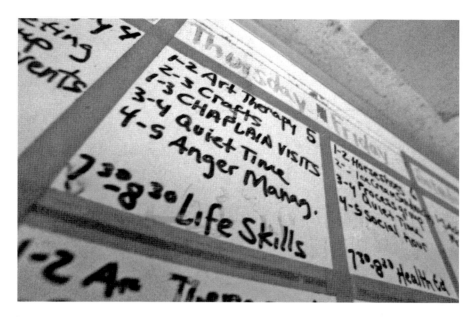

Ward schedule, secure unit. *Courtesy of author.*

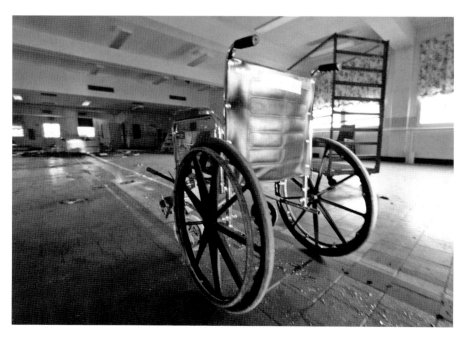

Patient wheelchair, secure unit. *Courtesy of author.*

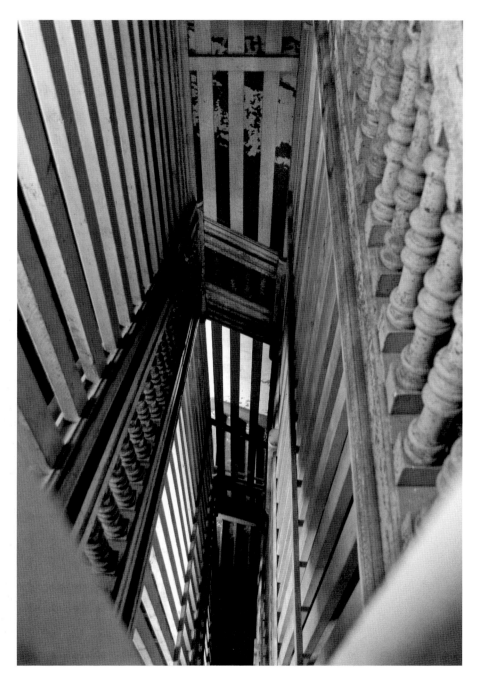

Administration stairway, Babcock. *Courtesy of author.*

11.
FOUR DECADES IN THE TRENCHES

It was a locked ward, and it was a threatening ward. People used to fight all day. We used to have to stop fights every thirty minutes.
—*Wilhelmina Rivers*

Over her forty-one-year career at the South Carolina State Hospital, Wilhelmina Rivers worked with just about every kind of psychiatric patient imaginable. As a mental health specialist (a position that was formerly known as a hospital aide), she saw it all—violence, racism, hate, fear, loyalty, love, laughter and tears. She took care of patients as old as eighty years old and others as young as four. She worked with some supervisors she liked and others that she described as "real mean." She cleaned up messes that would have made a goat gag and broke up more fights than she could count. She was bitten, cursed, spat on and smacked, and she was ultimately sent into an early retirement after a patient attack shredded her knee and left her back permanently damaged.

Yes, River's career on Bull Street was anything but easy, and it paid so modestly that she had another job at Holiday Inn. Yet despite the inherent challenges that came with her work in the mental health field, she still speaks of her four decades at the hospital with an unmistakable sense of pride, purpose and passion.

"A THREATENING WARD"

Rivers was still a teen when she headed to Bull Street looking for work. The year was 1975, and she'd just graduated from nearby Dreher High School. She got a job as a mental health specialist (MHS) and was responsible for bathing, dressing, feeding and caring for patients, and—perhaps most importantly—she was responsible for protecting the patients from themselves. Hers was an entry-level position that the administration normally hired young black women for during the 1970s and 1980s. "You wouldn't see a white person doing the job that we did," explained Rivers. "If a white person applied for a job as a mental health specialist, the supervisor would encourage them not to do that. They thought it was embarrassing to have whites as mental health specialists." Rivers was one of the thirteen MHSs assigned to Ward 118 in the Williams building. There were sixty-three female patients in there, about 70 percent of them black and most of them violent.

"It was a locked ward, and it was a threatening ward," said the retired MHS. "People used to fight all day. We used to have to stop fights every thirty minutes." But Rivers adapted quickly—she had to. During her first week on the job, a patient smacked Rivers while she was dressing her, and other women threw violent fits every time they were taken to the shower. For the especially unruly, there were three seclusion rooms on the ward; if anyone went into a rage, they were given a sedative and locked in one of them. On most occasions, it worked but not always. Rivers said there were incidents in which an employee would unlock the seclusion door after the allotted time, only to find the still enraged patient lunging right for them.

For a salary of about $400 per month, the MHSs were also entrusted with the unenviable duty of chasing and restraining patients who attempted to escape the grounds. "One time, I was chasing after a lady, and she got in a big green trashcan," Rivers recalled. "So, I went and got the trashcan and rolled her down the hill… back toward the campus until security came to help me." Rivers claimed patients would most often attempt to escape when they were being transported to their

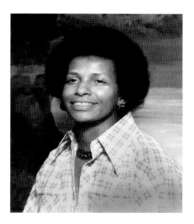

Mental health specialist Wilhelmina Rivers pictured in the 1970s. *Courtesy of Wilhelmina Rivers.*

hometowns for court hearings. A team of MHSs would accompany them to ensure they didn't evade custody. Back then, Rivers asserted, she was still young and in good shape and could usually catch any female patient who got a case of the happy feet.

COMMITMENT TO PATIENTS

Almost immediately after starting her career at the state hospital, Rivers took a strong liking to the patients of Ward 118 and developed a special affinity for the women who'd been there for many years. "I liked the older patients, because they were loyal to you," she explained. "They all had names for you, and you had to get used to all the names. If you resembled someone in their family, they would call you by that name, and you weren't going to change their mind. You would get so used to it that you would just answer to [that name]."

In the 1970s, state hospital patients enjoyed a lot more liberties and privileges than they did in the decades that followed. When Rivers started, MHSs would eat most of their meals in the same cafeteria as their patients. In addition, employees were allowed to bring off-campus food to their patients, and they could even take them off the hospital's grounds on a day pass.

> *When I first started working* [at the hospital], *I brought a patient home for Christmas.* [The patient] *had a sister who used to work there, but the sister left and never came back to see her. So, I took her out of there on Christmas and drove her around the town, sightseeing for a while. Then, I took her home for Christmas dinner and bought her a present.*

But as the deinstitutionalization movement gained steam and the DMH's budget shrunk, the institution's rules inevitably tightened, and staff members were no longer allowed to carry out such acts of compassion.

Bull Street employees didn't get many pay raises either—an institutional defect that created a huge turnover in nurses and MHSs during the hospital's final decades. With three children of her own to care for and a husband who also worked as an MHS, Rivers took a cleaning job at the nearby Holiday Inn on Assembly Street to supplement her income. Rivers's mother would watch over her kids while she clocked out from the hospital around 3:30 p.m. and headed straight to work at the hotel. Originally, she was supposed to get off work at the hotel at 7:00 p.m., but she said there were many evenings that her management would keep her there until 10:00 or 11:00 p.m. Indeed, nobody on Bull Street could ever question Rivers's work ethic or commitment to her patients, even if the price for her dedication was a stagnant salary and a hospital administration that was increasingly unaccommodating.

OTHER PATIENTS

Suffice it to say Rivers witnessed some wild incidents during her two decades working in the Williams building. She saw one patient give birth inside a seclusion room and another who was so obsessed with becoming a mother that she went to unimaginable extremes. "One of my patients always wanted a baby," recalled Rivers. "Well, she was getting a check-up one day, and the doctor saw a baby's head inside her. She told him the baby was coming, and he believed her, but it turned out to be a baby doll's head." If a patient died on the ward, Rivers claimed a team of MHSs had to pack their body's cavities and prepare it for the morgue—it was the part of the job she disliked the most.

After working with the women of Ward 118 for roughly twenty years, Rivers was moved to the hospital's back wards to work with men. "The men were much better behaved than the ladies," she said of the men she worked with for a half decade in the high-security Preston and Saunders buildings. "Some of them were respectful. If they liked you, they liked you, and they wouldn't let anybody hurt you."

Unfortunately, the same could not be said for the institution's teen patients, many of whom had been transferred to the William S. Hall Institute straight from the Department of Juvenile Justice (DJJ). Not only were these adolescents violent, but they were also almost impossible to control. As noted in Chapter 8, retired hospital public safety officers said they were often called to the Hall Institute when things got out of hand. "The teen patients would riot and everything. They would tear the ward up," said Alexander. "They would tear water fountains off the wall, toilets, anything they could destroy…They were real trouble, and they would escape regularly, because Hall Institute wasn't made for those types of patients."

Although Rivers's long career had left her battle-tested, she said nothing could have prepared her for the chaos and danger of working with troubled teens. "Oh, it was awful," she explained. "That was the worst ward I ever

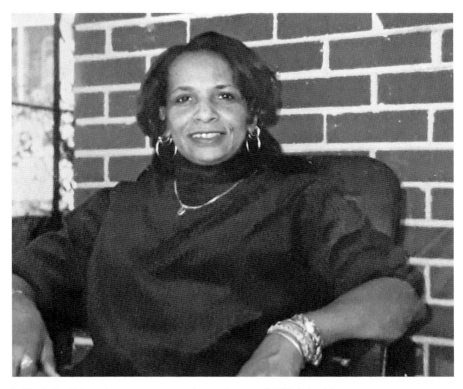

Wilhelmina Rivers in a more recent photo. *Courtesy of Wilhelmina Rivers.*

worked. They fought all the time. They were disrespectful. They weren't loyal. If they didn't get what they wanted, they'd flip on you. They were real bad. That was an awful job, right there."

Despite their bad behavior, Rivers did feel genuine compassion for the kids. In addition to suffering from mental illness, nearly all of them had endured physical abuse at the hands of adults and older children. It was standard practice for MHSs to read their patients' charts to get a better understanding of those they were caring for, and their histories were often rife with tales of abuse and cruelty. Just as the MHSs would accompany the adult patients to legal hearings, they also often escorted the hospital's adolescents to and from the courtroom. It was a sad and emotional experience for all involved. "They'd be crying, and we'd be crying with them, because they didn't know where they were going—[they just knew that] they weren't going home anymore," Rivers explained.

END OF AN ERA

The Hall Institute remained functional for many years after every other building on the Bull Street campus was boarded up and abandoned. In the final stage of her career, Rivers continued to work with the adolescents in the institute, who almost universally referred to her as Grandma. Over four decades after she'd started at the state hospital, her job was more dangerous than ever.

One day in 2016, she was monitoring a seventeen-year-old boy who'd earned a reputation for getting into fights. When staff members informed him that the skirmishes had temporarily cost him his video game privileges, the irate young man demanded to call his mother. Rivers got the phone and dialed the digits for him.

> *The number was busy, but I kept trying to dial it for him. He snatched the phone from me, and I tried to get it back. While I was doing that, he crossed his feet around my ankles and pushed me real hard. I fell and messed up two discs in my back and tore my meniscus. I had to have surgery on my knee and get treatment for my back. When I left that day, I never went back.*

Thus, her career, which spanned four decades, came to an inglorious end. Today, the sixty-three-year-old Rivers is retired and chooses to spend most of her time with her children and grandchildren. She lives in downtown Columbia on the corner of Liberty and Broad Streets, and on Friday nights, she has a good view of the firework show at Spirit Communications Park. That stadium, of course, stands as the centerpiece of the recent Bull Street redevelopment project, and it is within shouting distance of the Williams building, where Rivers spent the first two decades of her career. An unfortunate part of living so close to the campus is that Rivers often comes face-to-face with her former patients, who now wonder the streets with neither a home nor hope.

> *I never did, in my entire life, think* [the hospital] *was going to close. When they started putting patients out on the street, they didn't know where to go. I used to see some of the patients around my neighborhood.* [I saw] *one man* [whom] *I remembered from Building 1 at the State Hospital* [who] *had AIDS. The last time I saw him, he was drinking liquor, had a colostomy bag and didn't even know who he was. It was so sad to see him like that, because when we had him in Building 1, we had church on the ward for them to go to and gave them all kinds of activities to do.*

12

A SOCIAL WORKER REMEMBERS THE LATE 1970s

Some of the stuff I saw there was just unbelievable.
—Melton Francis

When Melton Francis went to his job interview at the South Carolina State Hospital, he made one crucial mistake: he left his pack of cigarettes visible in his shirt pocket. It wasn't that his interviewer cared that he smoked—in 1977, you could light up just about anywhere—it was that the patients who saw the cigarettes wanted them. Thus, Francis found himself the center of attention when he toured the female wards of the Babcock building after his interview. "It was a little unnerving for me, because there were two or three women in restraints, tied to the bed, and the others were walking around like zombies," he recalled. "They just started surrounding me—grabbing at my pants and grabbing at my pockets. It took two social workers and a couple of orderlies to get them away from me." When he returned to the administration office, Francis made one thing clear: if he was hired, he wanted to work in the male wards. They said they'd call him about the job in a week or two. Instead, they called him at 8:00 a.m. the next morning and told him that he had the job. So, Francis started his two-year stint as one of the hospital's few master-level social workers.

Francis's road to Bull Street had been a long one; after graduating from Spartanburg High School in 1967, he enrolled at Wofford College. However, his poor academic performance during his freshman year made him a prime

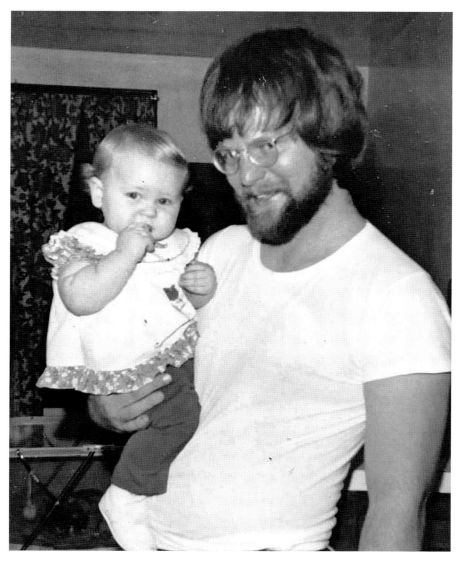

Former master social worker at South Carolina State Hospital Melton Francis. *Courtesy of Melton Francis.*

target of the U.S. draft board. Choosing to exercise the small amount of control he had over his fate, Francis enlisted in the air force and flew to Vietnam to work as an aircraft mechanic. Francis returned to the United States in 1969 and was back on the Wofford campus two years later. This time, he excelled academically and graduated in 1973. Francis married his wife, Lisa, the following year, and after struggling to find work, the couple decided to move to Columbia and enroll at the University of South Carolina, Francis in the graduate school and Lisa in an undergraduate program. In May 1977, Francis received a master's degree in social work, and he started his job at the state hospital the following month.

WORKING THE WARDS

Francis's office was on the same hall, in the central administration section of the colossal Babcock building, with the other high-level social workers. His usual caseload consisted of roughly twelve to eighteen patients.

> *I was the intake social worker for the admission ward on the men's side* [of Babcock]. *As patients would come into the facility, I would have to go back and talk to them before they were medicated, and* [I would] *get a feel for what was going on with them. After I talked to them, I would call their family and do a complete social history on them to find out what was going on with them at home.*

After that initial meeting, Francis would regularly check in with his patients throughout the course of their stay, which generally lasted between six weeks and six months. Typically, doctors would place patients in the admission ward for three to five days, then to a locked ward and, finally, to an open (or unlocked) ward before discharging them. "I was back on those wards every day, checking on those guys," he said. "Some of the stuff I saw there was just unbelievable."

One alarming incident Francis experienced was a rare group escape from one of the hospital's locked wards, which occurred just three weeks after Francis had started working at Bull Street.

> *I don't know how they did it, but they somehow knocked the bars and windows out on the second floor* [of Babcock]. *There were about eight to ten of them, and they all jumped out of those windows. One* [patient] *broke his ankle, and another one got bruised up real bad, so the two of them were just lying there. But the other six to eight…left the grounds.*

Twenty minutes after the escape, a fellow Bull Street social worker rounded up the unruly gaggle at the bus station just a few blocks away. "I was told anytime anybody [left] the hospital—whether they escaped or walked off the grounds or whatever—they always [went] to the bus station to catch a bus to go back home," Francis explained.

MOST MEMORABLE PATIENTS

Of the many patients with whom Francis worked, two men particularly stuck out to him. His first notable patient was a Charleston attorney who suffered from manic depression, which is now known as bipolar disorder. Francis said each time the lawyer sensed a manic episode coming on, he'd drive to Bull Street and commit himself.

> By the time we all met with him, he would be in a total manic state, and you really couldn't talk to him. He would just be going a mile a minute about antiques, about how he was going to sue for the release of every patient in the hospital, about how he was going to set up a practice in the hospital…It's funny, because every time he was there, the other patients would tell me they had a lawyer who was working to get them out.

Francis's other notable patient was a middle-aged African American, whom Francis described as "sophisticated" and "very outgoing." A dozen years before Francis met the man, he had killed his landlady but was declared "incompetent to stand trial." He was sent to the state hospital under the condition that he go before a judge every three months for a competency hearing. Like clockwork, the patient would start behaving strangely the week before the proceeding, talking to himself and reporting visual and auditory hallucinations.

> The court would always rule him unfit for trial, and then he would get back to the hospital and be fine. He told me, "It's a lot easier being here in the hospital than in jail. When I'm here, I can go outside, I can walk on the grounds when I want. I can go to the commissary. They take me on field trips. They take us to the movies now and then…In jail, I can't do any of that."

Francis also saw several patients admitted to the hospital for "alcohol-induced psychosis." Typically, these patients were fine once they sobered up and were usually released in a few weeks. The problem for them, of course, was staying sober once they were out. The retired social worker remembers one alcoholic who returned to the hospital drunk as a goat. The patient told the staff that he hadn't touched any liquor or beer but that he did take an occasional sip of Listerine mouth wash. His breath was fresh, but his blood alcohol concentration level was 0.35 percent, roughly four times the legal limit.

A REVOLVING DOOR

Of course, patients didn't need substance abuse problems to make return trips to Bull Street. Francis estimated that between 80 and 85 percent of the patients he worked with returned to the hospital, back in the grips of severe mental illness. He blamed two trends for that revolving door. The first was deinstitutionalization, which, by the time he arrived at the state hospital, was in full swing. As a result, the hospital's doctors were releasing patients prematurely. "They were wanting to get everybody either to a halfway house or back home," Francis recalled. "I thought it was a very bad idea." Francis claimed that the second contributor to so many readmissions was his patients' inability to purchase their medications once they were back in their communities.

> *The primary thing that I saw was that a lot of* [the patients] *were able to get an apartment and a job and everything, but they would end up back in the hospital, because they'd say they couldn't afford the apartment, food and their medication. So, they would let go of the medication, because they felt okay. It was a financial thing for most of them. They just couldn't afford it.*

Suffice it to say some such cases had tragic endings. One of Francis's patients returned to the hospital in a full-blown rage. The retired social worker described the man as "a giant," who was around 6 feet and 6 inches tall and weighed between 350 and 400 pounds. When staff members were unable to pacify or tranquilize him, they locked him in a seclusion room ("rubber room") naked so that he couldn't hang himself with an article of

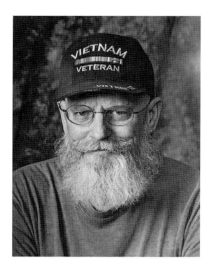

Melton Francis today. *Photo by Barney Tull.*

clothing. He committed suicide anyway. "[He] got on one side of the room, and he put his head down," Francis recalled. "He ran and just bashed his head into the door as hard as he could. It just crushed the vertebrae in his neck, and it killed him instantly, right there in that room."

The only other suicide that took place in Babcock during Francis's time occurred when a man in the admission ward somehow came into the possession of a web belt—the kind used in the military. "He crawled under his bed one night, put that belt around his neck, and he physically pulled that thing until it crushed his throat, and he died there underneath that bed," said Francis.

SALARIES AND CELEBRITY SIBLINGS

The 1970s were financially tough on Bull Street. In 1973, DMH director William S. Hall told the South Carolina Budget and Control Board that the hospital would lose its accreditation if they didn't double the amount of staff.[25] The hospital's financial situation remained dire even after its patient population fell to 1,922 by 1975, less than half its total a dozen years earlier.[26] "They had to fight for every penny they got," said Francis, who alleged there was a 100 percent turnover rate among the hospital's nurses while he was there. It's a staggering statistic, but at Bull Street, the jobs were tough, and the pay terrible. Even with a master's degree in social work, Francis earned just $700 per month, an amount that was grossly insufficient after he and Lisa welcomed their first child into the world. "If the pay had been better, I would have stayed there," he admitted. "The people working at the state hospital while I was there were pretty dedicated to our patients and wanted them to get the help they [needed] to succeed."

Two of Francis's best friends at the hospital even had famous siblings. Helen Danner, the hospital's chief of social work, was the older sister of actress Blythe Danner (from TV's *Will and Grace* and the film *Meet the*

Parents). Meanwhile, one of the hospital's psychologists, Mike Conroy, was the brother of bestselling author Pat Conroy (who wrote *The Prince of Tides* and *Lords of Discipline*). "I had no clue that Mike was his brother," Francis explained. "I was sitting in my office one day, and Mike walked in and threw a paperback copy of *The Great Santini* on my desk. He said, 'You need to read this book. It's about a marine pilot that is my dad.'" Francis even got to meet the man who inspired the famous novel, Colonel Donald Conroy, when he came to Babcock one day to pick his son up for lunch. Francis informed Conroy that he'd served overseas in the air force, and the two men spent several minutes talking about planes. Ironically, around the same time, Warner Bros. began shooting the film version of *Santini* in Beaufort, which starred Robert Duvall in the lead role and none other than Blythe Danner as his loyal but overmatched wife.

BACK TO THE AIR FORCE

Ultimately, Francis's salary on Bull Street just wasn't enough to support a family of three. After learning of his predicament, a friend of his from graduate school recommended that he return to the air force and gave him the number of a recruiter in Charlotte. The recruiter came to the state hospital to interview him, and within weeks, Francis was back in the air force. His pay went from $700 a month to almost $2,400. "You just can't say no to that," he admitted.

Francis climbed to the rank of captain by 1981 and moved to Kansas a decade later, when McConnel Air Force Base was leveled by a devastating string of tornadoes. He retired from the air force in 1995 but decided to stay in Kansas, living in the small town of Derby. After leaving the service, Francis spent the next seventeen years in social work, helping special-education kids in the Derby public school system. Today, Francis is fully retired and residing just a few miles from Wichita, a city with a growing homeless population. Seeing so many struggling souls living on the streets makes him lament the death of our nation's giant psychiatric hospitals. After all, from 1977 to 1979, he witnessed the curative powers of such places firsthand. "The people you now see on the street are the ones who used to seek inpatient treatment in the state hospital system," he explained. "I think that system offered a good alternative for a lot of people, especially the lower economic class. It gave them a safe place where they could get effective treatment."

13.
THE RARE VOLUNTEER

Every single one of [the patients] *had been abused in some way. It was shocking to me....Knowing the awful things they'd gone through was just another reason that I didn't want to quit and leave them.*
—*Robin Stancik*

I guess I was about twenty when I started. I was really idealistic, and I had no idea what went on." That's how Robin Stancik felt when she signed up to volunteer at the South Carolina State Hospital in 1983. In fact, Stancik had just graduated Columbia College (which she'd attended on a music scholarship) and was considering a career in music therapy when she first arrived at the gates of Bull Street. That idea didn't last long. Upon discovering that a juvenile patient had attacked and bitten the hospital's last music therapist, Stancik decided a full-time job at the hospital wasn't for her. Even after that discovery, though, the young Columbia native spent the next half decade volunteering to help the female patients hidden behind the institution's walls.

From the outset, the hospital's staff had no idea what to do with her, as a full-time volunteer was a rarity at Bull Street. Someone decided Stancik should start out working with the children in the William S. Hall Psychiatric Institute. Although she was only inside the Hall Institute for a few weeks, it was long enough for her to hear some truly horrifying stories. "Those kids... they didn't have a chance," recalled Stancik, who is now fifty-seven years old. "One kid had been tortured by his family. They'd done things like put him in the clothes dryer. His babysitter had burned him with cigarettes and killed the family pet in front of him. That kid was, like, six. Those kids were young, you know?"

Soon after her arrival, the hospital's administration decided Stancik's services would best be utilized in the Wilson building, which housed a ward for schizophrenic women. And though these patients were significantly different from the children she'd worked with in the Hall Institute, they'd suffered many of the same nauseating abuses. Stancik saw this damage with her own eyes when a hospital social worker gave her a couple dozen patient charts to read. "Every single one of [the patients] had been abused in some way," she explained. "It was shocking to me. I was young and bright-eyed and just didn't know that was how the world operated. Knowing the awful things they'd gone through was just another reason that I didn't want to quit and leave them."

So, for the next five years, Stancik dedicated one day and one night each week to caring for the ladies of the Wilson building. She would have spent more time with them had she not taken on a full-time job at the nearby Riverbanks Zoo. In any case, the hospital's administration gave the young volunteer freedom to do whatever she wanted on the ward. She spent most of her time just trying to comfort and entertain the patients, baking them cakes and playing cards with them. After a while, she even brought her own jambox to the ward to play the old funk music the patients favored. One patient, an African American lady in her fifties who went by the name Sweet Georgia Brown, would put on different wigs and dance to the music. "They just wanted people to spend time with them," reflected Stancik. "A lot of their families had just taken them there and left them, and they wanted to know somebody cared about them."

Indeed, the Wilson building was a lonely place to call home. Because the patients there suffered from severe schizophrenia, most of the women stood little chance of functioning in society. And since they were considered chronic long-term patients, nurses and doctors shunned them in order to work with those patients who had better chances of improvement and recovery. With no supervisors in the Wilson building to keep an eye on them, Stancik claimed the orderlies who worked there could be quite unpleasant. "They scoffed at the patients. They laughed at them a lot," she remembers. "They weren't nice. I saw acts of kindness from the activity therapist and the social worker, but I never saw any acts of kindness from the orderlies." One night, Stancik claimed the orderlies intentionally locked her inside the dayroom with the female patients and headed out

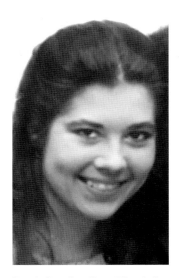

South Carolina State Hospital
volunteer Robin Stancik.
Courtesy of Robin Stancik.

to a Christmas party. The former volunteer said that incident was especially unnerving because the women were unpredictable and often fought among themselves. One day, a woman even hallucinated that an activity therapist was her cheating husband, and she "retaliated" by breaking a pool cue over his back. The therapist never returned to the state hospital. The fact that Stancik herself was never attacked in all her years of volunteering illustrates the rapport she enjoyed with the patients, and not just those in Wilson.

Toward the end of Stanick's stint at Bull Street, she was asked to help chaperone patients on off-campus field trips. One year, at the state fair, she tried to convince a patient, who'd never even heard of cotton candy, to try it. "She thought I was nuts," Stancik recalled. "She thought I was eating cloth or insulation or something." Though she couldn't comprehend why hospital officials would entrust a volunteer to chaperone patients at the state fair, Stancik fully understood the importance of getting the men and women away from the Bull Street campus from time to time. After all, behind the gates of the South Carolina State Hospital, patients remained mostly out of sight and out of mind. "Once I was outside the gates, I would feel like nobody knew or cared about the people in there," she said. "They were worried about these superficial things like football, while those people were just pushed out of everybody's eyesight so that no one had to look at them or think about them."

Stancik said she had no intention of staying at Bull Street as long as she did, but she felt obligated, because she was the only friend some of the women in the Wilson building had. "I just couldn't stop, because I loved them so much," she said. It wasn't until she got married and became pregnant that Stancik finally said goodbye to the hospital for good. By then, it was 1988 and America's deinstitutionalization movement was in full swing. The Wilson building was shuttered soon thereafter, and hundreds of the hospital's patients were moved to community mental health centers across the state. Though she never returned to Bull Street, Stancik often wondered about the fate of her old friends. Even today, they remain a fixture in her memory—they were teachers that provided Stanick with some of the most important lessons of her early adulthood. "They brought me a lot of happiness, and they made me understand a lot about life," she said. "They taught me not to jump to conclusions but to try to think [of] what people [may have gone] through [to make] them the way they are."

14.
A PATIENT'S BATTLE BACK FROM THE BRINK

It was an overdose, and it could have killed me. I forgot what it was, but they had to pump my stomach, and I ended up shutting down emotionally. I was at Baptist Hospital on the eighth floor for quite a while. I lost so much weight and was so depressed that they gave me ECT.
—Jan Wise

Usually, the symptoms of mental illness don't manifest themselves until a person reaches adolescence or early adulthood. But for Jan Wise, the writing was on the wall as far back as she can remember. "Even as a child, I had problems," she said. "I think back about times that I was reprimanded or had done something wrong. I would get in a closet and say that I wanted to kill myself or I wanted to die, and that's not normal for a child of six or seven [years of age]."

Born in 1955, Wise grew up in Cayce, a town just west of Columbia. During her early childhood years, Wise's parents tried to ignore the depression and diminished self-esteem they saw in their daughter. In the early 1960s, after all, the stigma surrounding mental illness was fierce, and treatment still rudimentary. During her teen years, Wise began self-medicating with drugs and alcohol, frequently using speed, marijuana and LSD. She admitted that she was impulsive and mischievous, and her parents and teachers dismissed her behavior as that of a wild teenager just looking for some fun. Then, when she was seventeen years old, Wise half-heartedly attempted suicide by swallowing a handful of antihistamine pills. Nothing much came of the incident, but her parents did send her to see a counselor at the First Baptist Church of West Columbia.

As a student at Winthrop College, Wise continued to party. "I had a great time. I stayed there a half-dozen years and majored in about five subjects," she explained. It was during this time that Wise spoke to a counselor at the Rock Hill college. The counselor suggested that she may have been suffering from bipolar disorder, which was then known as manic depression, and referred her to a psychiatrist in Charlotte, but Wise never went. Finally, as the 1980s dawned, Wise dropped out of school and moved to Charlotte, where she partied, met new people and took several odd jobs that came along. Wise even drove an ice cream truck for a day, but the incessant chime of "Pop Goes the Weasel" made that experience a short-lived one.

When she inevitably ran out of money, Wise returned to Cayce to live with her parents. At age twenty-seven, this was a cold and bitter taste of reality, and Wise's depression came crashing back down like a tidal wave. Her second suicide attempt, in 1982, was far more serious. "It was an overdose, and it could have killed me. I forgot what it was, but they had to pump my stomach, and I ended up shutting down emotionally," Wise recalled. "I was at Baptist Hospital on the eighth floor for quite a while. I lost so much weight and was so depressed that they gave me ECT [electroconvulsive therapy]."

Through her illness and treatment, Wise's mischievous streak remained alive and well. Once, a friend of Wise's snuck two beers up to her hospital room. When the nurses discovered them, they punished Wise by putting her in a straitjacket. A judge committed her to Baptist Hospital's psychiatric unit for another two months, but soon after she was released, she spiraled into another bout of crippling depression. This time, she was sent to the South Carolina State Hospital.

"A SAFE PLACE"

After checking into the Bull Street facility, Wise was placed in the William S. Hall Psychiatric Institute. Wise's memory of her time there remains foggy, but it proved to be a crucial first step in her recovery journey. "I guess Hall was a safe place for me," she said. "It kept me from being impulsive, and I had a good doctor. I think he was an intern from the university, and maybe once a week, they would take me to see him. That's the first time I learned anything about coping skills…from that nice doctor there."

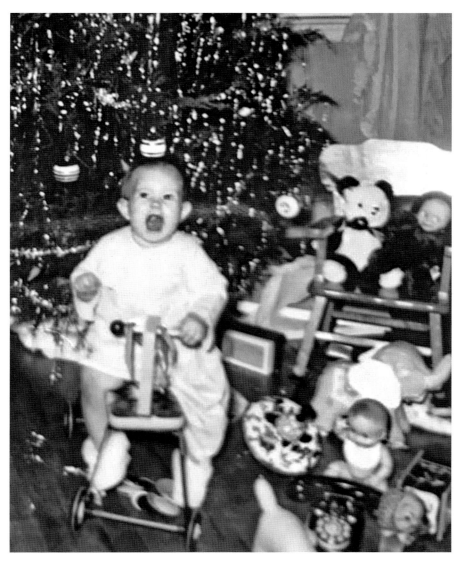

Baby photo of Jan Price, former patient at South Carolina State Hospital. *Courtesy of Jan Price.*

While she admitted that the Hall Institute seemed a bit overcrowded compared to the Baptist Hospital, Wise insisted that it certainly "wasn't a torture chamber" of any sort. She was placed in a ward with women suffering from a vast range of mental disorders and slept in a room with four to six other patients. Instead of recommending more ECT, her doctor prescribed lithium, an alkali metal that has helped stabilize bipolar patients since the middle of the twentieth century. At first, Wise had difficulty just getting out of bed, but the nurses coaxed her up each morning and prohibited her from sleeping during the day. Eventually, her depression began to wane, but the same cannot be said for her wicked streak. "I tried to make the best out of a bad situation, and I was kind of a mischievous patient at the time," she recalled. "I remember, one time, I bought some Tide [detergent] and put it in the fountain in the main lobby, and I got caught. I was mischievous—just a kid at heart—but they kept a good eye on me. They had to."

As a naturally social person, Wise bonded easily with other patients. After living on Bull Street for a couple of weeks, Wise earned a "yard card," a document that gave her the freedom to walk around the sweeping grounds of the state hospital's campus. On her walkabouts, she got to know several of Bull Street's permanent residents, patients who were deemed too sick to ever be released from the hospital. Wise would talk to them and take them candy and cigarettes. She said one elderly man she befriended had been a patient there for over two decades.

The only other time Wise was able to interact with male patients was during recreational excursions off campus. She laughed when she recalled one such field trip the patients took to see the 1983 horror movie *Christine*.

> We were sitting in the van, and I forget if it had something written on the side, but it was pretty obvious we were a group from the state hospital. We were stopped at a red light, and I remember someone in another car staring at us, so I pretended I was choking the guy sitting next to me. I think my humor kept me going through all of that.

"A MISSION FOR ME"

After six weeks at the state hospital, Wise was discharged and emerged with a new sense of stability and purpose. "What I've come to terms with now is that Jesus Christ had a mission for me in life," she explained. "Those suicide attempts were screams for help, but they could have killed me. There's a reason why I'm on this earth. My mission is to help people, to help children." With the aid of medication and the coping skills she acquired at the Hall Institute, Wise set about tackling life as a grown-up.

She enrolled at Midlands Technical College to boost her grade point average and later transferred to the University of South Carolina, where she earned her psychology degree in 1987. Significantly, she also said farewell to the booze and dope. "The combination of drinking and drugs wasn't a good one, with me being so impulsive and vulnerable," she reflected. "It was a danger for me to do that, and I finally learned the hard way."

So, Wise started her career working with children in the late 1980s. Her first job was with the Department of Juvenile Justice (DJJ), and she later found a position she loved, working with younger children at the Boys and Girls Club of the Midlands. Despite her fondness for the nonprofit foundation, she was eventually lured away by a teaching job that was closer to her home and offered a much higher salary. That position in Lexington School District 2 required her to work with emotionally disturbed seventh and eighth graders who'd been expelled from the county's public school system. Though Wise's intentions were admirable, it didn't take long for the inherent danger of the job to present itself.

When a classroom fight broke out between two of the students, she and another teacher attempted to intervene. One of the boys, who Wise insists was at least six feet tall and weighed two hundred pounds, threw her across the room, fracturing her back and ribs and damaging her spleen. Weeks later, when Wise had recovered enough to walk, she returned to the school at the urging of her supervisor. It was a mistake that would trigger a full-blown psychotic episode in Wise.

> *I went back* [to the school], *and this new kid, with a history of gun violence, looked at me and told me he was going to cap me. I had great fear that night and went back to school the next morning, and* [I] *got so upset that I went into a fetal position up under one of the other counselor's desks. She took me to Baptist Hospital.*

Despite the physical and psychological toll these two incidents took on Wise, there was, in fact, a silver lining to them. During her weeklong stint at Baptist Hospital, Wise's doctor put her on a new drug called Abilify. "Since then, I tell ya'…it's like a miracle how I've been able to function," she said.

"NOT A DEATH SENTENCE"

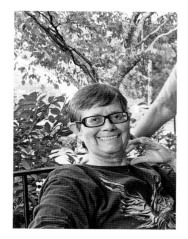

Jan Price today. *Courtesy of Jan Price.*

After supplementing her new medication with regular visits to a psychiatrist and therapist, Wise flourished. She returned to the Boys and Girls Club of the Midlands and took a job as a staff supervisor, working with seventy to ninety kids per day. For nine years, Wise worked with the Boys and Girls Club to improve the safety of and accountability for children between the ages of four and eleven. It was work that Wise described as "very rewarding," and she did it until she retired last summer to care for her mother full time.

Wise remains optimistic about her continued recovery and has learned how to handle the "intrusive thoughts" that used to rock her. As the following story from Wise illustrates, she is working to become an advocate for victims of mental illness. Soon, she envisions herself speaking to large groups and sharing her story of perseverance and courage.

> *I'm very upset about people with mental illnesses getting a bad rap, and I worry that, in the direction we are going politically,* [mental illness] *could become* [stigmatized] *once again. It does not have to be a death sentence. It does not have to control your life. A person has some control and responsibility. I think a lot of* [this control comes from] *learning coping skills and being educated about what your illness is. It's also very helpful to reach out to others, instead of just isolating* [yourself].

15.
DRIVE TOWARD DEINSTITUTIONALIZATION

What [doctors] *wanted to do was provide the education and training to the psychiatric residents in a controlled setting. So, what they did was pick and choose patients out of the state hospital population that covered a broad spectrum of illnesses and* [brought] *them over to Hall for training purposes. So, they basically used the state hospital as a pool for patients.*
—*Jack Balling*

In Jack Balling's three decades as the director of budgeting for the South Carolina Department of Mental Health (SCDMH), he got an insider's view of deinstitutionalization. The late twentieth-century movement, which entailed the gradual closure of large state mental hospitals in favor of smaller, community-based facilities and programs, forever changed the face of psychiatric treatment in America. Like hundreds of other hulking asylums that housed mental patients for well over a century, the South Carolina State Hospital now sits mostly abandoned, its buildings and grounds frozen in a Pompeii-like stillness.

Of course, the old campus in downtown Columbia was still pulsing with life when Balling first arrived there in August 1970. After graduating from the University of South Carolina with a degree in business, the Delaware native became an assistant hospital administrator at the William S. Hall Psychiatric Institute. The Hall Institute, which was named after the state commissioner of mental health at the time, was a teaching hospital used for conducting psychiatric research and training mental health personnel.

One of the institute's most significant functions was its psychiatric residency program, which was created in 1961 for physicians going into the psychiatric field of medicine. As a Hall Institute administrator, Balling got a firsthand look at some of its training programs.

What [doctors] *wanted to do was provide the education and training to the psychiatric residents in a controlled setting. So, what they did was pick and choose patients out of the state hospital population that covered a broad spectrum of illnesses and* [brought] *them over to Hall for training purposes. So, they basically used the state hospital as a pool for patients.*

Balling was promoted to the position of SCDMH director of budgeting in 1976 and moved into the department's new administrative building across the street from State Hospital. At that time, he estimated that there were roughly 3,000 patients on Bull Street's campus and another 3,000 on the Crafts-Farrow campus off Farrow Road. The late 1970s and early 1980s proved to be difficult for the old hospital, with budget cuts, staff shortages and deteriorating facilities creating a storm of controversy. In 1977, the Associated Press reported that, together, Bull Street and Crafts-Farrow needed 486 more nurses to match patient demand.[27] In 1981, the state hospital lost its national accreditation after failing to meet federal standards for the amount of nurses working there.[28] Balling said the demand for nurses was a constant problem for two reasons. First, there were few nurses that wanted to go into the psychiatric field, and second, the state hospital had a hard time keeping the nurses they did get. "State salaries weren't competitive with other local hospitals or even the VA hospital," said Balling. "If you hired somebody, the other hospitals would turn around and offer them $10,000 more, and it was just hard to compete."

CHANGE FINALLY CAME TO the beleaguered hospital in 1986, when Joseph Bevilacqua took over as the SCDMH director when Hall retired. Having already served as state mental health commissioner in Rhode Island and Virginia, Bevilacqua was a well-established champion of the deinstitutionalization movement. In fact, he'd even served with Virginia's Task Force on Deinstitutionalizationin 1978.[29]

[Bevilacqua] *came in right after the Justice Department* [controversy] *and had a great budget decision before him. He could have gone to the* *legislature and said he needed $20 million to hire new nurses and doctors that they needed* [at the two State Hospital campuses]. *Or, he could* [have invested] *in community programs to move folks out of the hospital. He chose the latter, because that was the trend of the time—deinstitutionalization.*

The former budgeting director said Bevilacqua spent his first six months as commissioner monitoring the state hospital system in its existing form. Then, he went to work, bringing in consultants from across the country and moving patients from Bull Street and Crafts-Farrow to community facilities and transitional living quarters. Balling asserted that the federal Medicaid program provided a significant stimulus for emptying state-run mental facilities.

Since its inception in 1965, Medicaid has had an exclusion policy which bars federal funding for patients between the ages of twenty-one and sixty-four admitted to an institution for mental disease (which was defined as any mental facility with more than sixteen beds). Since the state hospital obviously fit into this category, most of its patients were ineligible for Medicaid and had to rely completely on state funding for the round-the-clock care they received. The only logical way for the DMH to circumvent this exclusion policy was to move asylum patients either to nonmental facilities (nursing homes, general hospitals, et cetera) or to smaller community-based mental hospitals with less than sixteen beds. Once the patient was transitioned to one of these destinations, Medicaid was once again required to foot the bill, allowing state funds to go toward other patients and purposes. "Medicaid took care of a lot of budget problems," Balling recalled. "It allowed DMH to earn significantly more revenues for inpatient services while providing better care for these patients who were really in need of nursing home care."

Though Bevilacqua was hardly the first SCDMH administrator to tweak the system to secure Medicaid dollars, he was the first to virtually empty the state hospital in the process. "In the end, [Bevilacqua] stayed [at the hospital for] about ten years and did a lot of good things to force the issue [of funding]," said Balling. "By the time Bevilacqua left, we were down to about seven hundred patients."

Medicaid's role in the deinstitutionalization movement was a pivotal one. By 2001, Medicaid reportedly accounted for over a quarter of public mental health spending in the United States.[30] Although Balling's long stint with the DMH came to an end seven years ago, the sixty-four-year-old remains more

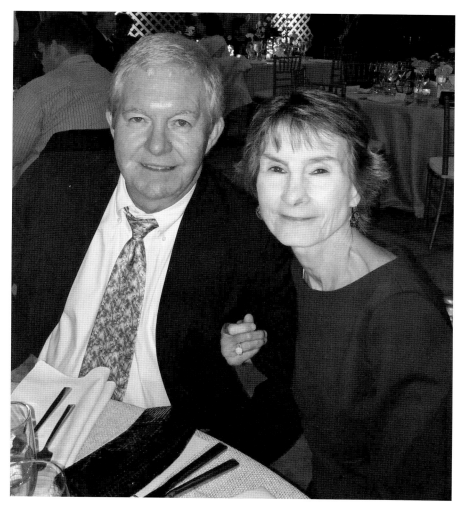

Jack Balling and wife, Stormy, today. *Courtesy of Jack Balling.*

active than ever in the mental health field. As the president of the South Carolina chapter of the National Alliance on Mental Illness (NAMI), he spends his days recruiting volunteers and organizing events for the nonprofit advocacy group, which has gone from a humble $10,000 operation to an $80,000 agency in just a few years.[31]

16.
THE WHISTLEBLOWER[32]

[The] *State Hospital has always been the repository of humanity. That's always been my perception. What doesn't fit anywhere else fits there.*
—*Jack Luadzers*

FROM PRISONERS TO PATIENTS

Missouri psychologist Jack Luadzers didn't come to South Carolina in the 1980s to work at the state hospital; he came to work with sex offenders at the Kirkland Correctional Institute. Having trained under groundbreaking sex criminologist Barbara Schwartz, he was hired by the Kirkland Correctional Institute to design treatment programs for sex offenders in the maximum-security Columbia prison. His work there culminated in the opening of the Gilliam Psychiatric Center, a facility inside Kirkland where sex criminals were housed, evaluated and treated. However, when government funding for Gilliam's program began to evaporate, the psychologist went to Bull Street to design a new predator program at the state hospital. "[At the state hospital], I ended up with a very well-defined, tight group of sexually aggressive people that were drawn from all over the system—people who kind of rose to the surface as having extreme, sexually aggressive traits," he said. "These were people who had never been adjudicated—some with easily thirty-three to forty victims—who had never been caught."

In his fifteen years of working at Bull Street, Luadzers saw his fair share of neglect, filth, violence and overcrowding. He saw the hospital's dayroom chairs stained with excrement and patients with toenails that were so long they clacked the floor when they walked. "[The] state hospital has always been the repository of humanity," he claimed. "That's always been my perception. What doesn't fit anywhere else fits there." Luadzers also said he witnessed the hospital's administration employ some shadowy tactics, such as a scheme to dupe national accrediting agencies that inspected the hospital.

> *Little did the accreditors know that the patients with really bad things in their chart, like too many restraints and other things that* [were] *against the law,…we would put them on a bus with their charts and transfer them for a couple of days* [to the Crafts-Farrow campus seven miles away]. *Then, they'd come back* [when the accrediting body had left].

"THESE WERE PREDATORS"

While Luadzers found the patients on Bull Street to be challenging, he was immediately impressed with the therapists and doctors there. "When I first started, I met some of the most qualified, intelligent and superb clinicians that I ever met in my career," he said. "They were dedicated people. You can't train people to work with this population [of sexual predators]. It takes very unique people to understand what you're dealing with." But the rapid movement toward deinstitutionalization did a number on the hospital, and as the patients disappeared so did the staff. Luadzers said that of the thirty-two psychologists who were on the payroll when he started, only three remained by the time he was named the hospital's chief psychologist.

Joseph Bevilacqua's resignation in 1996 only seemed to deepen the hospital's budget cuts and accelerate the transfer of its patients to community-based psychiatric programs. Dr. George Gintoli took over as the DMH director in 2000, and the department faced a significant budget cut in his first two years. In fact, the Associated Press reported in 2002 that the SCDMH lost around $50 million in state and federal dollars and had to eliminate 882 employees between the years of 1999 and 2001. Struggling to cut spending anywhere he could, Luadzers alleged that the director began unloading dangerous patients in 2001.

He was hired specifically to take out the institution and close state hospital...I repeatedly explained to him and outlined that we [had] *extraordinarily dangerous patients. I went to the commission. I was writing notes that clearly delineated these patients as a clear and present dangers to all populations. These were predators.*

The therapist said a clear distinction exists between common sex offenders and genuine sexual predators, in that "predators live to offend." He said true predators will marry, find jobs and choose neighborhoods all with the intent of getting closer to child victims. He said predators will oftentimes even have children for the sole purpose of molesting them. The psychologist claimed that, while the majority of sex offenders are responsive to psychiatric treatment, sexual predators "really cannot be stopped, because [the impulse to hunt] is so ingrained in their circuit board."

"AN OPEN LETTER"

Luadzers was on his way to the airport, planning to fly to San Francisco for a work conference, when he got an infuriating phone call. At the other end of the phone was a personal friend, who informed him that the state hospital had quietly dumped two of his most dangerous patients into the City of Sumter.

[These patients] *were in these community care homes with no supervision.* [The hospital officials] *had thinned the charts so that they didn't even reflect the fact that they were pedophiles. I didn't go to San Francisco—I couldn't. I drove to my house in Folly Beach and wrote my manifesto—an open letter to every newspaper in the state.*

That letter, which accused the hospital of releasing dangerous patients back into society as a result of the drastic DMH budget cuts, was picked up by the Associated Press, whose story appeared in papers everywhere on May 5, 2001.[33] The allegations Luadzers made in the letter raised millions of eyebrows across the state and the nation. Despite Gintoli's declaration that "no one at the hospital is let go before they are ready to be,"[34] South Carolina attorney general Charlie Condon ordered a SLED investigation of the hospital's release policies. Luadzers said little came of the investigation, however, because the agency gave the DMH "plenty of time to cover their tracks." In the days that followed the letter's publication, the psychologist asserted that the department once again altered the charts of the two patients and sent police to Sumter to find them.

Though South Carolina citizens applauded the psychologist for making an ethical stand and for putting their safety ahead of his own job security, Luadzers said he received a predictably cooler reception from his department officials. "I was hoisted on everybody's shoulders except the administration's," he recalled. "The commission acted like I'd never spoken to them [about the concerns I voiced in the letter]." A few months later, Luadzers retired from the hospital and filed a lawsuit against the DMH, alleging that they had demoted him from chief psychologist to human services coordinator as a form of punishment and to prevent him from reviewing patient records. The case was settled out of court soon thereafter, bringing a final sense of closure to the psychologist's sixteen-year run at the Bull Street institution.

Luadzers continues to be a vocal critic of the deinstitutionalization movement, which he believes landed the mentally ill in prisons, shelters and emergency rooms, instead of the state hospitals that were equipped to treat and shelter them.

> *Most of my former patients are now inmates at Lee Correctional Center (a maximum-security prison thirty miles west of Florence). I know that for a fact, because I've visited them there, and they are treated horribly. It's a terrible thing. Two-thirds of our homeless are mentally ill, wandering around. I predicted back in 1991 that emergency rooms [were] going to be completely inundated with mental patients, and they are. [During] the first cold snap, you're going to see emergency rooms completely jammed.*

17.
THE ACTIVITY THERAPIST

I'll never forget the eyes of one of the patients who had never seen the ocean. The awe on her face when she felt the water on her toes was amazing. She was probably in her fifties and had been at the hospital pretty much her entire life.
—*Kim Grant*

The first time Kim Grant took a tour of the South Carolina State Hospital, she wanted to run far away. It was January 1979, and she was a senior at the University of Georgia. She'd driven for three hours to interview for a student internship at Bull Street that March, but a tour of the gargantuan Babcock building had left her shaken. The building's stench was thick as she walked past patients lying on the floor, moaning and reaching toward her with tobacco-burned fingers. When she completed her interview, she ran across busy Elmwood Avenue to a nearby payphone and called her father in Thomson, Georgia. Crying and frantic, she explained that maybe the facility wasn't the right place for her after all. Certainly, Grant would never have guessed that she'd spend the next twenty-two years working at Bull Street and loving every day of it.

"NO COMPLAINTS"

Despite her initial trepidation, Grant got the internship and worked in the state hospital's activity therapy program from March to June that year. While

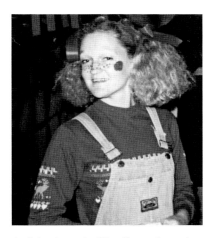

Activity therapist Kim Grant dressed as a clown. *Courtesy of Kim Grant.*

assisting an experienced therapist, Grant spent her days with female patients in the Allan and Saunders buildings at the back of the campus. She helped organize cookouts, exercise classes and gardening sessions for the patients, and she frequently took them across the campus to Bennett Auditorium, where they could enjoy movies, dances and other leisure activities. "I feel I had a good internship and learned a lot from so many therapists," said Grant.

Indeed, that three-month stint transformed Grant's perspective of the hospital from horrific to hopeful, and she committed herself to a career there. When Grant's internship concluded, she rushed back to Athens to collect her degree in therapeutic recreation before returning to Columbia a week later as a full-time activity therapist. "I started [at Bull Street on] June 22, 1979, and my starting salary was $10,736," she recalled. "I thought I was rich, I really did. I had no complaints."

Grant also had no complaints about her job requirements, which included working with older men in the Allan building, who hailed from the state's Pee Dee region. One of Grant's first projects with these patients was a garden that was just outside the ward. That summer, they grew squash, cucumbers and tomatoes and sold them by the pound to employees across the hospital's campus. By August, they'd raised about ninety dollars, which Grant spent taking them to lunch at the Hilltop Restaurant off Saint Andrews Road. Shortly thereafter, the hospital administration decided to build a large greenhouse at the back of the Bull Street campus.

"A NEW WAY TO BE OBSERVED"

As the 1980s dawned at the South Carolina State Hospital, the institution's forty to forty-five full-time activity therapists continued to play a pivotal role in patient treatment. For one thing, patients genuinely enjoyed the leisure activities Grant and her colleagues created for them. On campus, there were regular birthday parties, miniature golf tournaments, talent shows, fashion programs, dances, movies and cookouts. The therapists also produced programs for every holiday, including an annual Christmas play and what Grant described as "the best Halloween carnival ever." Grant recalled of the carnival, "The Benet gym was transformed with walls of colorful streamers to make booths for games that were created and made by the therapists. We had a wheel of fortune, a turkey shoot, a cakewalk, skeetball and putt-putt just to name a few."

Indeed, the Benet Auditorium was, what Grant called, "a crown jewel" for therapists. It offered a large gym, a clubroom with pool tables, TVs and board games, and a full-service library with newspapers, books and magazines. The auditorium's lower level was a designated clinical space for ceramics, crafts, fitness, woodworking and music. It allowed therapists to teach and observe specialized referral groups.

But as much as the patients enjoyed the Benet Auditorium, it was the off-campus recreational trips they seemed to love most. Grant got her commercial driver's license (CDL) so she could drive her patients out to fast-food restaurants, discount stores, the flea market and barbecues at nearby Sesquicentennial State Park. On occasion, the patients were taken on longer excursions that required more supervision and planning—fishing tournaments at Fort Jackson, strawberry picking at Cottle Farms and trips to the zoo and state fair. Grant even started a bowling league for her patients; she took them to the bowling alley every week and threw an awards banquet with trophies at the end of every season. Occasionally, activity therapists would take patients on all-day trips to Santee State Park, and once, Grant even took her patients all the way to Myrtle Beach. Even after all these decades, this is a trip that remains etched in her memory. "I'll never forget the eyes of one of the patients who had never seen the ocean," she reflected. "The awe on her face when she felt the water on her toes was amazing. She was probably in her fifties and had been at the hospital pretty much her entire life."

One trip to Sesquicentennial State Park proved unforgettable for a much different reason.

One of the saddest things I ever saw while working [for the hospital] *happened at a picnic at the park. We had a patient that left the group and walked into a pond and drowned. They found him late that afternoon. That was a sad day for all of us. Probably six to seven months before that, that same patient had tried to escape but security had found him and brought him back. I always wondered if he just lost hope for going home.*

Grant claimed that this incident afforded therapists and leadership the opportunity to change accountability policies on field trips, ensuring that patients were better monitored and protected. After all, everyone at the state hospital realized that off-campus excursions proved critical when gauging patient behavior.

> *I think our service provided the patients with a new way to be observed. Their behavior on the unit might be completely different from what they would display in the community off the unit. It gave* [the patients] *a chance to interact with each other and* [staff members] *in a more relaxed environment, where I felt we could really get to know them and what was bothering them.*

Because of the unique insight they were able to provide, activity therapists were an integral part of the treatment teams assigned to each patient. They worked in conjunction with the other members of their teams—nurses, social workers, doctors and psychologists—to conduct a monthly review of each patient. Teams would score each patient, in areas such as daily living, hygiene and group attendance, in order to determine their eligibility for off-campus trips.

"WE WORK IN THEIR HOME"

Just as Grant found her first tour of Babcock deeply unsettling, her first elevator ride in the building also unnerved her. This event occurred on the first day of her internship while she was taking her suitcase to her fourth-floor bedroom. Before the doors could close, a peculiar looking patient got in behind her.

> *He had an obvious limp and a platform shoe on one foot. He was chanting a song, snapping his fingers and peering at me above his sunglasses. I did not think I would see the fourth floor that day, but when the elevator stopped on the third floor, he exited to his ward, gave me a wink and hobbled off. The next day, I described him to my new coworkers, who told me that everyone knew him. He was harmless and sort of the king of the campus. I guess it was at that moment that I decided not to fear these patients but to get to know them, love them and provide activities for them.*

Years later, Grant kept a quotation on her office wall that read, "The patients don't come to our office. We work in their home." Indeed, for most of her patients, the state hospital had been their home for years. Some had even lived there most of their adult lives, and a few of them were there from the day she arrived until the day the hospital closed in the early 2000s. Grant said that some of her patients felt like peers, while others felt like her own children. She even worked on the weekends to complete her paperwork so that she could have more time with the patients during the week. "I just had a good rapport with the patients," she said. "I never had one try to attack me. I think the key to that was that I always tried to treat patients the way I wanted to be treated. I always tried to give them a concrete answer, not a vague answer. I used real concrete thinking with them, and I think that helped." There is also no doubt that Grant's position as an activity therapist helped her, because she represented a fun diversion from the hospital's mundane daily routine. "[Activities] gave [the patients] something to look forward to. [They] gave them hope," she said. "I really felt blessed, because every day, I put my feet on the floor and my mind was already thinking about what I was going to do that day."

Teaming with other activity therapists, Grant worked constantly to come up with fresh activity ideas. Perhaps their single biggest accomplishment was starting a Family Day, where patients could enjoy food and fellowship with their family members. A lot of effort, time and forethought went into the event, which took place on a Saturday in May. The afternoon's entertainment was held in the Benet Auditorium and varied year to year. During one Family Day, Grant and her colleagues put on a production of *Let's Make a Deal*. Another year, they produced a play for the occasion. By all accounts, the event was a major success and eventually attracted over three hundred family members to the hospital in a single day.

"IT'S ALMOST LIKE WE WENT BACKWARDS"

By the 1990s America's deinstitutionalization movement was in full swing, and the South Carolina State Hospital was downsizing rapidly. The Gibbes, Lieber, Wilson, Babcock, Parker and Laborde buildings were all emptied, and the patient population, which had numbered over 3,000 when Grant arrived, had dropped to about 530.[35] Despite this declining trend, Grant said that Bull Street had made significant strides when it came to patient

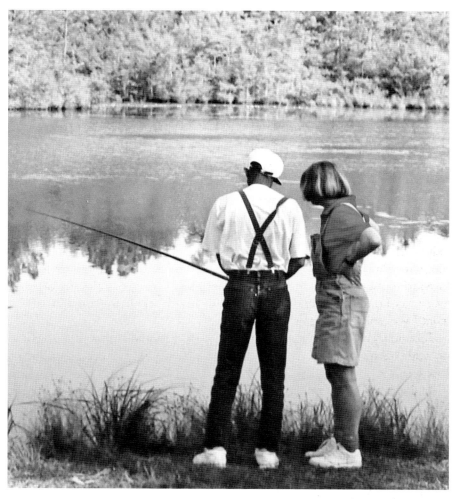

Kim Grant and a patient fishing during an off-campus field trip. *Courtesy of Kim Grant.*

treatment and overall campus environment. "There was an emphasis on updating furniture to a more home-like look," she explained. "Bright colors and fabrics replaced metal chairs and vinyl coverings. Window treatments, blinds and fresh paint made the wards more welcoming, and patients wore nicer clothing."

But even with these overdue improvements, time was not on the state hospital's side. The institution began to shut down in 2001, and by the following year, all of the adult patients were gone. For Grant, this was a sad moment in South Carolina's mental health history. "I don't think you could have told me that place would ever close until it did," she said. "I thought it was probably the best program that could have existed for the treatment of the mentally ill. When it closed, it took a big chunk of treatment out, and it's almost like we went backwards. I felt like we weren't making progress anymore."

In 2001, the DMH moved its forensics program from Bull Street to its Crafts-Farrow campus just a few miles away. Grant was offered a job as the supervisor of the unit and immediately accepted. Most of the hospital's therapists, equipment and supplies were relocated to Crafts-Farrow. Until Grant's retirement, she was able to continue working as an activity therapist, taking patients on field trips and preparing them for their eventual return to public life. Although Crafts-Farrow was more overcrowded and less picturesque than Bull Street, Grant continued to enjoy her work. "I loved forensics, because the patients were eager for new activities," she said. "They loved to do things, and I think the psychiatrists [at Crafts-Farrow] did a great job stabilizing them with medicine. They could just do a lot more and were a fun group of people to work with—very respectful, very nice and very appreciative."

The fact that the patients were so well behaved illustrates just how far psychotropic medication had come since Grant's arrival at Bull Street. The forensic patients had, after all, committed serious crimes but had been ruled mentally unfit for trial or not guilty by reason of insanity. While many continued to judge them for their deeds, Grant made a concerted effort to abstain from judgment, knowing these patients suffered from grave mental illnesses. "To me, [the patients] were there for mental health treatment," she said. "I never looked at it like I was treating them for their criminal behavior. I was not. I just decided I was there to treat them for their mental health issues and provide for them what I could [so that they could live the] best lives that we could give them while they were there."

Grant said there were close to two hundred patients in the state's forensics program, and she knew almost all of them by name. In 2017, Grant finally retired after working for the DMH for nearly four decades. These days, Grant lives in Columbia and continues to lament the premature closing of the Bull Street hospital, where she spent some of her best years. "I think we closed the best place for the patients to be," she said. "I feel like a lot of patients did actually end up on the street. I went through downtown Columbia about six months ago, and I saw one of my old patients lying on the sidewalk by Main Street. A woman was trying to get him up so the police wouldn't come."

18.
A ROOKIE NURSE IN BYRNES

I had another lady come up and give me a big hug, and the next thing I knew, her teeth were in my shoulder. The family had come to visit, and they thought that I was abusing her, because she was covered in blood. Well, it was my blood.
—*Rachel Bricco*

E very morning, a twenty-one-year-old Rachel Bricco would get off the city bus at 2100 Bull Street and walk toward the hospital's guardhouse. After the security officer waved her through, she would take a left at the gargantuan Babcock building, walk past the Chapel of Hope and take another right at the sprawling Williams building. She would then walk through the parking lot and into Byrnes Medical Center, the urgent-care facility for the patients of the South Carolina State Hospital and inmates of the Central Correctional Institute (CCI).

Bricco started working at the Bull Street facility shortly after earning her nursing degree in 1984. While she was already working full time on the oncology ward at the nearby Richland Memorial Hospital, she took a daily 7:00 a.m. to 3 p.m. shift at the State Hospital to supplement her income. "Like with anything new, I was a little apprehensive," she remembers. "But the head nurse on the floor took me under her wing and introduced me to the patients. They were quite interesting. I wished the first one [I saw] a good morning and got hit up with a string of expletives, but she was really a sweet lady and we later became good friends."

During Bricco's year-and-a-half stint at Byrnes, she saw it all—from suicide attempts and attacks on nurses to the intake of death-row inmates and patients chasing imaginary chickens down hallways. However, most of her memories are fond ones, as she deeply enjoyed working with the patients and hospital staff. "Even with me being there in a temporary capacity, they were very welcoming," she said of her fellow nurses. "They were very helpful and instructional. They seemed like family."

The Greenville native worked primarily on the second floor of Byrnes, which, at that time, served as the hospital's surgical unit. Bricco said the first and third floors of Byrnes were used for urgent care, while the fourth functioned as a tuberculosis ward. The fifth floor of Byrnes was a lock-down unit, where mentally ill prisoners were treated and evaluated. One day, Bricco even got to see four policemen escort the notorious serial killer Donald "Pee-Wee" Gaskins through the building and onto an elevator bound for the fifth floor. "[He] was scary—very scary," Bricco recalled of the man who allegedly killed over one hundred people and was one of the last inmates to die in the state's electric chair.

Since Bricco didn't work on the fifth floor, she was mostly able to avoid the inmates and, instead, work with patients she mostly found interesting, kind and fun. She started at the bottom of the hospital's totem pole—bathing, feeding and transporting patients—and then graduated to handle documentation and the administration of medication. The career nurse said the use of tranquilizers and antipsychotics like Thorazine, Haldol and Meloril was commonplace at Bull Street, and she said straightjackets, vests and ankle restraints were used on especially unruly patients.

She said she was physically attacked five times during her eighteen-month career at Bull Street. Once, a male patient slapped her when she tried to get him out of bed for range-of-motion therapy. During another incident, a very small female patient somehow managed to pick her up and throw her across the dayroom. She also told the story of a patient who bit her.

> I had another lady come up and give me a big hug, and the next thing I knew, her teeth were in my shoulder. The family had come to visit, and they thought that I was abusing her, because she was covered in blood. Well, it was my blood. That took a long time to get straightened out, but it did get straightened out.

Obviously, working as a nurse in a state hospital wasn't for the faint of heart. Bricco said it wasn't uncommon to see injured nurses head

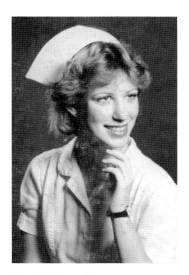

Rachel Bricco (former nurse at South Carolina State Hospital). *Courtesy of Rachel Bricco.*

to the Byrnes basement to receive stitches or tetanus shots before heading back up to resume their shifts. But more troubling to Bricco than the threat of physical violence was the prospect of her patients' lives being hijacked by mental illness. One time, she claimed she saw an eighteen-year-old girl come through Byrnes that resembled the possessed girl in the film *The Exorcist*. "She had stepped out in front of a car, and that's how she had broken both [of her] legs," Bricco recalled. "Her mother had gotten ill and was unable to manage her medication, so she had been without her lithium and antipsychotics. Once [state hospital doctors] got her medicine regulated, she was the sweetest young lady you would ever want to meet. But for days, she was *The Exorcist* girl reincarnated."

That young woman was lucky. Not only did she survive the collision with a car, but she was also able to recover and leave the hospital soon thereafter. At that time, most of the patients living at Bull Street weren't so fortunate. One case of a beautiful, young Ph.D. candidate still haunts Bricco to this day.

> *The first time I saw her, she was catatonic. The next time she came into* [Byrnes], *she had infected scratches where she had been trying to claw her eyes and everything out. We had no clue as to what was transpiring—a normal, healthy lady just gone…The last time I saw her, she was heavily medicated, had to be restrained, part of one eye was gone and she was severely disfigured.*

There was certainly no shortage of memorable patients and grisly episodes at Byrnes. Once, Bricco warned a man in the hall to clean up after himself before she read in his chart that he had set his house on fire and killed his wife and three children. Another time, she was wrapping the gangrenous foot of a patient, when the dressing got hung on one of the woman's toes. "It just snapped off like a twig, and she just looked down at me and said, 'Broke my toe off, did ya'?'"

Eventually, the South Carolina State Hospital was able to hire more full-time nurses and eliminate most of its part-time positions. In 1985, Bricco's stint on Bull Street came to an end, and she headed to Florence to manage a temporary staffing agency. Eventually, she returned to Greenville to be closer to her family and took a job at Oakmont Nursing Centers, where she found her niche working with geriatric patients.

Bricco said her short but eventful stint at Byrnes taught her lessons that proved invaluable later in her nursing career. "It was always interesting and very educational," she said. "Even though that was early on in my nursing career, there were things that I took from there that I used twenty years later." Among the most critical lessons she learned was that inactivity was detrimental to the mental health of patients. She also learned that standard methods of treatment weren't effective for everybody. "I found out that, instead of trying to strap somebody down who was walking and pacing, if I handed them a rag, they would wipe the doorframes," she said. "We had less behavioral problems when we gave [the patients] productive activities to do." Significantly, when Bricco was the manager of the Alzheimer's unit at Greenville's Brighton Gardens years later, she was able to reduce the rate of psychotropic tranquilizer use from 75 percent of the population to 17 percent by simply substituting productive activities for behavior modification.

19.
HER FAVORITE JOB

Of all the jobs I've had in my lifetime—and I've had a few—that was my favorite and the most fun.
—*Loretta Smith*

About six and a half miles northeast of the Bull Street gates stands the deteriorating campus of the Crafts-Farrow State Hospital. Used for decades to treat the state's mentally ill African American population,[36] the facility became a geriatric mental facility when the Bull Street campus was integrated in the mid-1960s. It's tough to imagine a bleaker place to start a career, yet that was where eighteen-year-old Loretta Fouche Smith took her first full-time job as a nurse's aide in the fall of 1975. "That was a real sad place—very sad," Smith said. "I worked on a closed ward, and I saw some things that really upset me, because I was young and new."

Each day at 7:00 a.m., Smith would unlock a heavy metal door with a skeleton key and walk through a stench of urine that took her breath away. She'd continue down the ward's hallway, through a grim chorus of wails and moaning, until she could hear patients shuffling their feet, a signature side effect of the drug Thorazine. Smith asserted that Crafts-Farrow was so strapped for nurses that the aides occasionally had to dispense medicine to patients. "One thing I [realized while] working in the field was that the people who cared the most were often the first to leave, because their hearts just couldn't handle it," she said. "In order to stay, you had to become somewhat callous to certain things."

After a year, Smith was tired of Crafts-Farrow and applied for a better job at the state hospital. She was only nineteen years old at the time, and she went to the interview wearing acid-washed jeans. Despite, or perhaps because of her casual attire, she landed a job in the asylum's recreation department as a therapy aide. "I think I got it because I was young and energetic and played guitar," she said.

HER FAVORITE JOB

As soon as she arrived on the Bull Street campus, Smith was blown away by the beauty and apparent serenity of the grounds. "It was park-like. There were benches everywhere, and [the campus had] fabulous trees," she recalled. "The patients were walking around and feeding birds and squirrels. It was very tranquil and peaceful. I just thought it was quiet and lovely, and the buildings were beautiful." This sense of excitement and hope was a welcome contrast to the despair and stagnation Smith witnessed at Crafts-Farrow. Of course, working in the recreation department was a lot more fun than being a nurses' aide. Smith worked in Bennet Auditorium, a facility near the front of the campus that offered patients access to a grand piano, basketball goals, pool tables, foosball and a host of other leisure activities.

"Of all the jobs I've had in my lifetime—and I've had a few—that was my favorite and the most fun," said Smith. Indeed, the new post offered its share of diversity. Smith and the recreational therapists she worked with gave cooking classes to patients, taught them crafts, played pool with them and performed music for their entertainment—and that was just during the daytime. At night, the auditorium hosted bigger attractions, like dances, plays and movie screenings. Smith said one of her duties was keeping patients from getting too intimate with one another during dances.

We tried not to have slow dances, because that could cause problems. But sometimes, patients didn't care if it was a slow dance or not, they would get physical. Well, they taught me how to break in if that happened and say, "Do you mind if I have this dance?" We actually had a technique to break that kind of thing up in a polite way.

Smith claimed it wasn't uncommon to have as many as 150 patients at the "open-ward" dances. The events at Bennet Auditorium were classified either

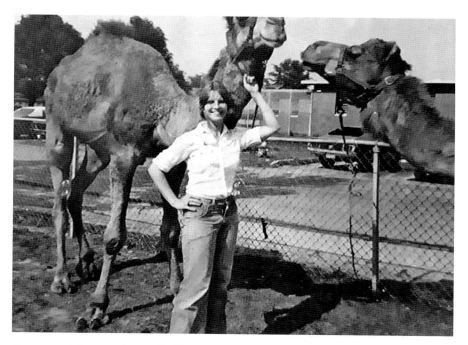

Recreational therapist Loretta Smith at a state hospital circus. *Courtesy of Loretta Smith.*

as "open ward" or "closed ward" functions. The more stable patients, who lived on open wards, were free to roam the campus and enjoy more privileges than their closed-ward counterparts, who were never allowed outside unless they were being transported in a large group. The latter were, generally, also more medicated, and thus less active and involved at recreational events. Closed-ward events required more security and closer monitoring so that patients didn't hurt themselves. In addition, only open-ward patients could use the auditorium during daytime hours.

In any case, dance nights and movie nights were the two most popular evenings of the week. The hospital had a huge popcorn machine for movies and booked a local band to play music at the dances. Disco was all the rage at the time, but Smith said the patients went especially wild when the band played the Steve Miller hit "Jet Airliner." One of the things Smith remembers most about working on Bull Street is having to go pick patients up for events in "the green machine," a full-sized 1960s-era school bus that had been painted green. Even though she didn't have a commercial driver's license, she drove patients to events that were both on and off campus.

REMEMBERING PATIENTS

While the job forced Smith to work with patients in large groups, it also afforded her plenty of time to get to know patients individually. She recalled one patient named Bill, who could play the grand piano with the skill of a concert pianist. Inevitably, however, his trademark perfectionism would ruin any enjoyment his talents provided him.

> *He used to play so well that it would draw me out of the office to listen. Then, he would hit one wrong note and slam the keyboard, storm off the stage, where the piano was housed, and stomp out of the auditorium, slamming the door and muttering obscenities as he left. I remember him so well. It was such a waste that he sought perfection to that point.*

Smith's saddest memory from her eighteen-month-stint at the hospital is of a young deaf patient who was only a couple of years older than her. He would often come to the auditorium during the day and try to help Smith with her sign language. One Friday, the patient was especially jubilant, because for the first time in many months, he was expecting a visitor over the weekend.

> *He was excited, and we were excited for him. It was a big deal. But when I came back to work on Monday, we couldn't find him. Well, what happened was, his visitor did not show up, and he became very angry. He started throwing things, and all they knew to do was drug him. The next time I saw him, he was completely out of it…catatonic, drooling…It was bad, because he was a young man—vibrant, coherent, seemed to be mentally healthy. That was a bad situation. That was very sad.*

After a year and a half, Smith left the state hospital for a job as a counselor with the State Department of Youth Services. While she was there, Smith worked in a dorm with sixteen- and seventeen-year-old boys who were undergoing evaluations after their arrests. It was a dangerous job, as some of the boys had committed violent crimes. But by using the social and interpersonal skills she'd acquired during her Bull Street tenure, Smith was able to remain safe and work effectively with the at-risk youths for the next three years.

After retiring from a three-decade career as an insurance underwriter, Smith now spends most of her time helping others on a volunteer basis.

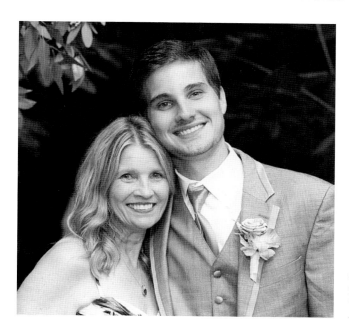

Smith today with her youngest son, Patrick Gilmore. *Courtesy of Loretta Smith.*

She teaches an after-school art class for kids, and as a Blue Star mother (her oldest son, Adam, is a captain in the air force), she also provides art therapy to veterans struggling with PTSD. "If you think about it, the arts speak to you when nothing else can," she explained. "People can express themselves in the arts freely when they can't anywhere else." Thus, four decades after she went to Bull Street as a nineteen-year-old in acid-washed jeans, Smith continues to employ the attributes and lessons she gained while working in the state hospital as a recreational therapy aide. "It was my favorite job," she said. "I learned about empathy. I learned that everybody has something they are dealing with. You don't get through this world without having to battle something, and I learned that there. It was a good training ground for life."

20.
A TEEN ON BULL STREET

I challenge anybody to go to Columbia Area Mental Health and try to get somebody admitted. These days, there is no mental health help, and I'll say that to anybody. You cannot get mental health help in South Carolina.
—*Bill Fort*

Before Alcoholics Anonymous (AA) popped up in every American town and addiction treatment centers became commonplace, alcoholics frequently poured into the South Carolina State Hospital. Though afflicted men and women weren't "mentally ill" by conventional medical standards, their reckless consumption of liquor caused them to behave in deviant, destructive and often unlawful ways. Their loved ones would take them to Bull Street as a last resort. When Bill Fort was just seventeen years old, he dropped out of Columbia High School and started working intake full time at the state hospital. He had no problem getting a job as a psychiatric aide, as there wasn't exactly a line of people waiting to get their hands dirty and take orders from nurses for eighty dollars per week. Fort, who is now sixty-seven, explained, "I did everything, from mopping floors and making beds to cleaning, restraining and escorting patients."

Having grown up in Columbia, Fort admitted he arrived at the job intimidated by all the stories and myths he'd heard about the hospital. For a while, in fact, he didn't think he was cut out for it. "My first few days there, I was sick to my stomach," he said. "That smell, the atmosphere…I didn't think I was going to be able to do it. But after the first week, I just fell in love

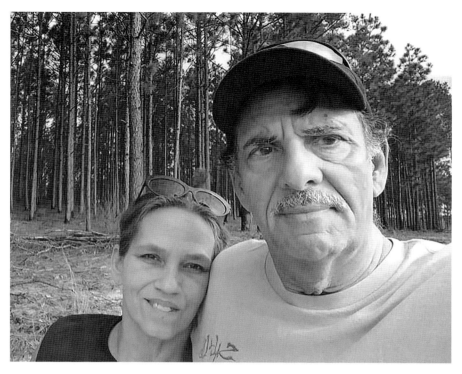

Bill Fort (former mental health specialist who worked on the State Hospital's admissions ward) pictured with his wife, Kay. *Courtesy of Bill Fort.*

with it. [The staff] got to be like family. We realized we were taking care of people that really needed us, and we did save a lot of people's lives."

Fort worked on the first floor of the Williams building, where patients of all types were admitted and held for a mandatory thirty-day observation period. The first two floors of the large brick structure were designated for female patients, and the top two wards were reserved for males. Fort estimated that about three out of every four patients he worked with were alcoholics. According to Fort, this was usually how his patients were admitted: family members would show up in the lobby with an intoxicated relative who didn't necessarily know they were being committed. After an interview and assessment process, the patient would be placed in a wheelchair and transported to a locked patient ward. If they became disruptive, they would be locked in a seclusion room and injected with a heavy sedative. If they were especially resistant, they would be sent to the tougher, more secure building at the back of the campus.

Fort claimed that, back then, the state hospital didn't really have a program in place for alcoholics; they were simply kept away from booze and given adequate food and rest. Most recovered their health and reason during the initial thirty-day observation period and were released. While patients were detoxing, it was Fort's job to monitor them and check their vitals to make sure they didn't have a stroke or go into delirium tremens (DTs). If they did begin to show symptoms of these conditions, they were administered immediate medical attention. Fort's job did have its perks, however, as the eighteen-year-old was allowed to participate in recreational activities, like playing cards with patients and reading to them. The job kept him busy, and he found it fulfilling to watch his patients progress from alcoholic despair to hope. "I liked the feeling of helping people," he explained. "I saw people come in, and I saw them go out. I saw a big difference after the thirty to sixty days that somebody was there."

Fort also enjoyed his coworkers. "The medical staff was very caring. They were good people," he claimed. "They wanted to do what was best for the patient. Everybody was real busy, and everybody had a job to do. There wasn't any time for any infighting or anything like that."

DESCENT AND REDEMPTION

After witnessing the devastation of alcoholism on a daily basis, it seems ironic that Fort succumbed to his own addiction while working on Bull Street, but the disease is cunning, baffling and powerful, and in 1969, recreational experimentation with narcotics was escalating. Fort said he began hanging out with the wrong crowd and smoking marijuana, which later progressed to taking opiates. He started shooting heroin and lost control of his life. No longer able to work, Fort walked away from his job at the state hospital, only to return months later as a patient. He spent six weeks inside of the Hall Institute for substance abuse treatment. But, just eighteen years old, he wasn't ready to go clean quite yet. He continued using drugs and was busted several times for simple possession. Finally, he violated his probation and was sent first to Columbia's maximum-security Central Correctional Institute (CCI) and then to Manning Correctional Institution (another maximum-security prison in Columbia). When Fort was incarcerated, he was nineteen years old and weighed less than 120 pounds but what seemed like the end of his road ultimately proved to be a new start.

First, Fort learned how to box, which improved his health, self-esteem and standing in the dangerous inmate community. "I had wrecked my health by age nineteen," he explained. "Boxing forces you to stay in shape. You can't halfway do it, or you'll get hurt. When the punches start coming, you have to move." More importantly, Fort returned to academics by first earning his GED and then by entering a college program that the South Carolina Department of Corrections (SCDOC) had established with the University of South Carolina. Three times a week, the prison bussed inmates across town to CCI for their classes. Without any drugs or a job to distract him, Fort excelled. "I owe a lot to the SCDOC for guiding me through obtaining a GED and beginning college," he said. "I'm living proof that corrections does work if done right."

Merle Haggard may have sung about turning twenty-one in prison, but Fort really did turn twenty while locked up at Manning. He still remembers his mother bringing a birthday cake to the visitation area there. When he was finally released after serving time for a year and a half, the young man stayed focused and drug free and earned his bachelor's degree in psychology from the University of South Carolina before working as a clerk in several area hotels. When that career path grew stale, Fort headed down to Florida to study motorcycle mechanics. He made his way to Key West, where he worked on mopeds for $7 per hour. While he was there, one man offered him $150 to come to Miami and box four rounds. Another offered him quite a bit more to smuggle drugs into Belize. Fort declined both opportunities, choosing instead to stay on the straight and narrow, and he returned to Columbia in 1982.

Three months later, he took a job as an employment counselor at a job agency on Calhoun Street, where he was once again able to work face to face with people and help them daily. For the first time in over a dozen years, he had a job he really enjoyed, and he kept it until his retirement in 2013.

THE COST OF DEINSTITUTIONALIZATION

Today, Fort admits his prison stint probably saved his life. "If I hadn't gotten locked up, I'd have never taken the GED, I'd have never taken the college boards, and I would have never enrolled at USC," he said. Eighteen months locked away from society may seem like a lot, but Fort said he needed that amount of time to reflect on his life and recover from his addiction. That personal lesson affirmed what Fort had observed while working on Bull Street. Alcoholics and addicts need adequate time away from society to make a new start in life. "You have to have a place where people can go for some time," he explained. "Time is what's going to heal them. If they just go somewhere to detox for a week or so, it's just going to give them enough time to work up a good thirst."

Fort said he witnessed this truth again a few years ago when his older brother died from the effects of alcoholism. Fort remains convinced that his brother would still be alive today if he had been able to go somewhere like the state hospital for thirty to sixty days. It's the primary reason he laments the closing of the Bull Street campus—there are no longer any public institutions where South Carolinians can get help for their addictions and mental illnesses. "I challenge anybody to go to Columbia Area Mental Health and try to get somebody admitted," he said. "These days, there is no mental health help, and I'll say that to anybody. You cannot get mental health help in South Carolina."

Fort remembers feeling the beginning of the tidal shift in mental health care when he was working in the Williams building in 1969. "At the time, in our state legislature, public sentiment went to deinstitutionalizing patients," he explained. "I think it was mostly proposed by the legislature to save money. I don't know how it happened, but all those services got defunded, and they don't exist anymore." Indeed, research shows that the state hospital's patient population fell from over 6,000 in 1967 to under 1,900 by 1975.[37] By 1986, there were fewer than 700 patients at the state hospital.[38]

Fort blames stories like Ken Kesey's *One Flew Over the Cuckoo's Nest* (1962) for vilifying state hospitals and perpetuating the deinstitutionalization movement. He said he never met any Nurse Ratchets during his time on Bull Street, just employees who cared about their patients and wanted to help them. "It was a wonderful facility, and when I was there, I knew we were doing good work," he said. "We could still be doing it now, but it's just gone away. That's why defunding and deinstitutionalizing mental health is one of the worst things to ever happen to South Carolina."

NOTES

1. Christopher Payne, *Asylum: Inside the Closed World of State Mental Hospitals* (Cambridge, MA: MIT Press, 2009).
2. Diana Garnett, Stephanie Gray and Kayla Halberg, "The Story: An Historical Narrative of the South Carolina State Hospital at Bull Street," Digitizing Bull Street, www.digitalussouth.org.
3. Garnett, Gray and Halberg, "Story: An Historical Narrative."
4. This story was written in 2010. In 2019, I attempted to locate Harris without success. I was told, however, that he remains alive and well.
5. James C. Kinard, "Number One Problem," *Aiken Standard and Review*, March 13, 1961, A4.
6. South Carolina Department of Archives and History, *State Department of Mental Health Annual Reports 1958–2000* (Box 3, Series 190002).
7. Peter McCandless, *Moonlight, Magnolias & Madness: Insanity in South Carolina from the Colonial Period to the Progressive Era* (Chapel Hill: University of North Carolina Press, 1996), 135.
8. Ibid., 218.
9. I wrote this story in December 2010. Elbert Metze passed away on October 22, 2015, at the age of ninety-four. Gertude passed away as I was working on this book in the summer of 2019; she was ninety-six.
10. It is possible that this is the same patient discussed in depth in the third chapter of this book.
11. Garnett, Gray and Halberg, "Story: An Historical Narrative."
12. Kinard, "Number One Problem."

13. Garnett, Gray and Halberg, "Story: An Historical Narrative."
14. I wrote this story in the summer of 2013. Today, six years later, Summers is eighty-five years old and still living in the Midlands.
15. Tom Summers, *Hunkering Down: My Story in Four Decades of CPE* (Columbia, SC: Edisto Press, 2000).
16. Ibid.
17. Ibid.
18. "Prosecutor Expects More Indictments," *Aiken Standard*, August 9, 1984.
19. South Carolina Department of Archives and History, *State Department of Mental Health Annual Reports 1958–2000* (Box 3, Series 190002).
20. Garnett, Gray and Halberg, "Story: An Historical Narrative."
21. "Aiken Citizens Hear About Mental Health," *Aiken Standard and Review*, December 8, 1959.
22. Garnett, Gray and Halberg, "Story: An Historical Narrative."
23. Doris A. Fuller et al., "Going, Going, Gone: Trends and Consequences of Eliminating State Psychiatric Beds, 2016," *Treatment Advocacy Center* (2016).
24. South Carolina Department of Archives and History, *State Department of Mental Health Annual Reports 1958–2000* (Box 3, Series 190002).
25. "SC Mental Health Department Runs Risk of Losing Funds," *Aiken Standard*, September 5, 1973, 4B.
26. South Carolina Department of Archives and History, *State Department of Mental Health Annual Reports 1958–2000* (Box 3, Series 190002).
27. "Funds Sought," *Florence Morning News*, September 21, 1977, 2A.
28. "State Hospital Decision Appealed," *Aiken Standard*, March 19, 1980, 3B.
29. "Virginia Official Top Candidate for State Job," *Aiken Standard*, October 5, 1985, 8B.
30. Richard G. Frank and Sherry Glied, "Changes in Mental Health Financing Since 1971: Implications for Policymakers and Patients," *Health Affairs*, May 1, 2006.
31. This story was written in October 2010. As of June 2019, Balling remains in Columbia and is still active in the state's NAMI chapter.
32. This story was written in 2010. I was unable to track down Luadzers in 2019, but a relative of his recently informed me that he was alive, well and living in another state.
33. "Psychologist Says Potentially Dangerous Patients Discharged from the State Mental Health Hospital," *Aiken Standard*, May 5, 2001, 4B.
34. "Psychologist Who Said State Released Dangerous Mental Patients Sues Over His Demotion," *Aiken Standard*, September 27, 2001, 8A.

35. South Carolina Department of Archives and History, *State Department of Mental Health Annual Reports 1958–2000* (Box 3, Series 190002).

36. Garnett, Gray and Halberg, "Story: An Historical Narrative."

37. South Carolina Department of Archives and History, *State Department of Mental Health Annual Reports 1958–2000* (Box 3, Series 190002).

38. South Carolina Department of Archives and History, *State Department of Mental Health Annual Reports 1958–2000* (Box 3, Series 190002).

INDEX

N

National Alliance on Mental Illness (NAMI) 9, 13, 40, 127, 160
Not Guilty by Reason of Insanity (NGRI) 15, 63, 76, 77, 138

O

open wards 109, 145
overcrowding 14, 53, 56, 58, 69, 120, 129, 138

P

Parker, Phil 15, 60, 61, 62, 63, 65, 66, 67
patient population 27, 29, 46, 58, 65, 71, 112, 124, 125, 136, 142, 143, 152
pregnancy 26, 32, 33, 57, 59, 116
Preston building 44, 45, 63, 104
prostitution 65
psychiatrists 14, 18, 48, 59, 76, 119, 123, 138

R

recreational therapy 133, 144, 147
restraints 19, 24, 26, 44, 61, 63, 102, 107, 129, 140, 141, 148
Rivers, Wilhelmina 101, 102, 103, 104, 105, 106

S

salary 60, 102, 104, 113, 122, 133
Saunders building 12, 14, 29, 44, 46, 61, 63, 104, 133
schizophrenia 15, 18, 31, 115
seclusion 44, 58, 61, 63, 73, 102, 104, 111, 149
Skipper, Helen 68, 69, 70, 71, 72, 73, 74

Smith, Loretta 15, 143, 144, 145, 146, 147
social work 15, 16, 75, 76, 77, 78, 107, 109, 110, 111, 112, 113, 115, 135
South Carolina Law Enforcement Division (SLED) 62, 130
Stanick, Robin 116, 117
straightjacket 16, 140
student nurse 14, 26
substance abuse 62, 78, 111, 150
suicide 14, 15, 19, 27, 44, 65, 112, 118, 119, 121, 140
Summers, Tom 13, 35, 36, 37, 38, 39, 40, 41, 154

T

Talley building 57, 58

U

understaffing 14, 24, 58, 69, 75
University of South Carolina 15, 51, 53, 75, 109, 122, 124, 151

W

Westbury, Ruth 42, 43, 44, 45, 46, 47
Williams building 24, 25, 53, 69, 71, 73, 102, 104, 106, 139, 149, 152
Wilson building 69, 115, 116
Wise, Jan 15, 118, 119, 120, 121, 122, 123

Y

yard card 76, 121

ABOUT THE AUTHOR

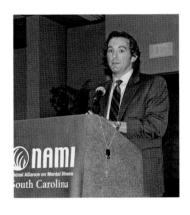

For nearly two decades, William Buchheit has worked as a journalist in Upstate South Carolina. He has won dozens of South Carolina Press Association Awards and was named the 2011 Reporter of the Year by South Carolina's chapter of the National Alliance on Mental Illness (NAMI). In recent years, he has become a part-time college English instructor and acclaimed wildlife photographer, whose photos of great white sharks have been published by *National Geographic* and the Smithsonian. *The South Carolina State Hospital: Bull Street Stories* is his first book. He lives in Greer, South Carolina.